DIABETIC SNACK & APPETIZER COOKBOOK

Mary Jane Finsand

□ □ □

Foreword by James D. Healy,
M.D., F.A.A.P.

 Sterling Publishing Co., Inc.   New York

EDITED BY LAUREL ORNITZ

RECIPE CONSULTANT: CAROL TIFFANY

Library of Congress Cataloging-in-Publication Data

Finsand, Mary Jane.
    Diabetic snack & appetizer cookbook.

    Includes index.
    1. Diabetes—Diet therapy—Recipes. 2. Snack foods.
3. Cookery (Appetizers) I. Title. II. Title: Diabetic snack and appetizer cookbook.
RC662.F567   1987   641.5′6314   87-10249
ISBN 0-8069-6558-4
ISBN 0-8069-6560-6 (pbk.)

Copyright © 1987 by Mary Jane Finsand
Published by Sterling Publishing Co., Inc.
Two Park Avenue, New York, N.Y. 10016
Distributed in Canada by Oak Tree Press Ltd.
% Canadian Manda Group, P.O. Box 920, Station U
Toronto, Ontario, Canada M8Z 5P9
Distributed in the United Kingdom by Blandford Press
Link House, West Street, Poole, Dorset BH15 1LL, England
Distributed in Australia by Capricorn Ltd.
P.O. Box 665, Lane Cove NSW 2066
Manufactured in the United States of America
All rights reserved

Contents

Foreword

The *Diabetic Snack & Appetizer Cookbook* is another excellent resource Mary Jane Finsand has added to her collection of fine diabetic cookbooks. In this book, Mary Jane shows how snacks can be tasty, nutritious treats that are very appropriate for diabetics.

I am sure you will find the *Diabetic Snack & Appetizer Cookbook* an invaluable resource book for your kitchen. The book includes calorie, carbohydrate, fat, and exchange information for each individual recipe, as well as information on brand-named prepared foods. Both conventional and metric measurements are listed, and there is a special section of fun-to-make-yourself recipes for children.

I commend Mary Jane for writing this book, which complements the series. She has made it much easier to plan a sensible, deliberate diet that diabetics and nondiabetics alike can live with and enjoy.

James D. Healy, M.D., F.A.A.P.

Preface

Snacking has become part of our everyday lives. But do you remember when your mother warned you that eating snacks between meals would spoil your appetite? Times have changed! Balanced snacks throughout the day are now regarded as helpful in controlling appetite and making weight loss easier for everyone.

For a person with insulin-dependent diabetes, between-meal and bedtime snacks can be a balance for the peak times of insulin and physical activity. In noninsulin-dependent diabetes, smaller meals with between-meal snacks can spread out the daily calories to make the body's insulin work better and help stabilize blood sugars.

Diabetes education can help you learn more about the relationship and balance between food, activity, and insulin. People with diabetes can then incorporate this information into their individual lifestyles.

Darlene K. Duke, RN
Diabetes Facilitator

Hattie M. Middleton, RN
Nutrition Facilitator

Covenant Medical Center
Waterloo, Iowa

Introduction

Snacking. . . . Most people think it's slightly sinful or at best self-indulgent, but as you probably know, snacks are a must in a diabetic's diet. Snacks, or more specifically small meals in between meals, help keep your blood-sugar level up where it should be.

Methods of testing and caring for diabetics have improved in recent years. If you follow your diet counselor and doctor's instructions, you can abate many of the more difficult and frustrating situations.

Diabetic children can be particularly difficult when it comes to their snacks. For this reason, I have included a small cookbook of snacks that is especially designed for children to use and enjoy. Allowing them to prepare some of their own snacks should increase their awareness of the value of snacks, instilling in them a habit that must be continued throughout their lives.

So that you can make nourishing snacks easily, I have included a snack-pantry list in the book, right before the recipes. Keeping a supply of the right products on hand should be helpful in your self-monitoring.

I hope the recipes in this book will bring joy and good eating to you and your family.

Using the Recipes— Conversion Guides

Read the recipes carefully. Then assemble all equipment and ingredients. Use standard measuring equipment (whether metric or customary), and be sure to measure accurately. Remember, these recipes are good for everyone, not just the diabetic.

Customary Terms

t.	teaspoon	qt.	quart
T.	tablespoon	oz.	ounce
c.	cup	lb.	pound
pkg.	package	°F	degrees Fahrenheit
pt.	pint	in.	inch

Metric Symbols

mL	millilitre	°C	degrees Celsius
L	litre	mm	millimetre
g	gram	cm	centimetre
kg	kilogram		

Conversion Guide for Cooking Pans and Casseroles

Customary	Metric
1 qt.	1 L
2 qt.	2 L
3 qt.	3 L

Oven-Cooking Guides

Fahrenheit °F	Oven Heat	Celsius °C
250–275°	very slow	120–135°
300–325°	slow	150–165°
350–375°	moderate	175–190°
400–425°	hot	200–220°
450–475°	very hot	230–245°
475–500°	hottest	250–290°

Use this candy-thermometer guide to test for doneness:

Fahrenheit °F	Test		Celsius °C
230–234°	Syrup:	Thread	100–112°
234–240°	Fondant/Fudge:	Soft Ball	112–115°
244–248°	Caramels:	Firm Ball	118–120°
250–266°	Marshmallows:	Hard Ball	121–130°
270–290°	Taffy:	Soft Crack	132–143°
300–310°	Brittle:	Hard Crack	149–154°

Guide to Approximate Equivalents

Customary				Metric	
Ounces Pounds	Cups	Tablespoons	Teaspoons	Millilitres	Grams Kilograms
			¼ t.	1 mL	1g
			½ t.	2 mL	
			1 t.	5 mL	
			2 t.	10 mL	
½ oz.		1 T.	3 t.	15 mL	15 g
1 oz.		2 T.	6 t.	30 mL	30 g
2 oz.	¼ c.	4 T.	12 t.	60 mL	
4 oz.	½ c.	8 T.	24 t.	125 mL	
8 oz.	1 c.	16 T.	48 t.	250 mL	
2.2 lb.					1 kg

Keep in mind that this guide does not show exact conversions, but it can be used in a general way for food measurement.

Guide to Baking-Pan Sizes

Customary	Metric	Holds	Holds (Metric)
8-in. pie	20-cm pie	2 c.	600 mL
9-in. pie	23-cm pie	1 qt.	1 L
10-in. pie	25-cm pie	1¼ qt.	1.3 L
8-in. round	20-cm round	1 qt.	1 L
9-in. round	23-cm round	1½ qt.	1.5 L
8-in. square	20-cm square	2 qt.	2 L
9-in. square	23-cm square	2½ qt.	2.5 L
9 × 5 × 2 loaf	23 × 13 × 5 cm (loaf)	2 qt.	2 L
9-in. tube	23-cm tube	3 qt.	3 L
10-in. tube	25-cm tube	3 qt.	3 L
10-in. Bundt	25-cm Bundt	3 qt.	3 L
9 × 5 in.	23 × 13 cm	1½ qt.	1.5 L
10 × 6 in.	25 × 16 cm	3½ qt.	3.5 L
11 × 7 in.	27 × 17 cm	3½ qt.	3.5 L
13 × 9 × 2 in.	33 × 23 × 5 cm	3½ qt.	3.5 L
14 × 10 in.	36 × 25 cm	cookie tin	
15½ × 10½ × 1 in.	39 × 25 × 3 cm	jelly roll	

Snack Pantry

Having a few items on your shelves or in your freezer can eliminate a lot of hassle when it comes to making snacks. Even though you can't always keep a full supply of every item you might want to use, you can store the ingredients you use the most and are most likely to run out of. At the end of this book, you will find a list of ready-to-eat snacks and small meal items from various food manufacturers, which should also be helpful.

Items You Might Want On Hand

Crackers, of different varieties
Soups, of different varieties
Small canned fruits, in their own juices
Small canned vegetables
Bouillon cubes
Small or individual frozen pizzas

*Noodles or pastas, of different varieties
†Rice, of different varieties
Dried Fruits
Dietetic Puddings and Gelatins
Spices and herbs
The usual dairy, dried, or fresh products

---

*Dry noodles or pastas can be kept on the pantry shelf, but you can freeze homemade in small bags. If you want to freeze cooked noodles, cook until al dente. Cooked noodles or other pastas do not freeze very well, however, unless they are in a prepared dish or meal.

†I always keep cooked white, brown, and wild rice in the freezer. To cook and freeze: Bring a large pot of lightly salted water to boiling. Even with raw white rice, you should use more water than you would normally use for steaming. Add rice to the boiling water, and then add a small amount of vegetable oil. Stir; then reduce heat (if cooking raw white rice on an electric stove, you can turn the burner off) and cook until al dente. Check after about 10 minutes. Wild rice will take longer. Do not overcook. When you can "cut" a rice grain with your finger, it is cooked enough. Immediately, pour rice into strainer and run cold water over it. Transfer rice to a cold bath. Change cold water several times to stop the rice from cooking. Turn rice back into strainer and allow any excess water to drain out. Flip rice with a fork. At this point you can either package it in serving or exchange sizes in small Zip-loc freezer bags, or turn rice out onto a pastry cloth to further remove any excess water and then package it. If you like a nutty flavor, try toasting the rice on a cookie sheet in the oven for just a few minutes until lightly browned.

Beverages

Pineapple-Grape Juice

2 c.	pineapple juice	500 mL
1½ c.	white grape juice	375 mL
¼ c.	lemon juice	60 mL

Combine ingredients and chill.

Yield: 3¾ c. (940 mL) or 8 servings
Exchange, 1 serving: 1½ fruit
Calories, 1 serving: 60
Carbohydrates, 1 serving: 16

Spiced Cranberry-Apple Juice

½ c.	water	125 mL
1	cinnamon stick, broken	1
¼ t.	nutmeg	1 mL
¼ t.	grated orange peel	1 mL
2 c.	cranberry-juice cocktail	500 mL
1 c.	apple juice	250 mL
1 T.	lemon juice	15 mL

Combine water, cinnamon-stick pieces, nutmeg, and orange peel in small saucepan. Heat to boiling. Boil 3 minutes. Remove from heat; then allow to cool to room temperature. Remove cinnamon pieces. Combine juices and spiced water. Chill thoroughly or serve hot.

Yield: 3¼ c. (810 mL) or 6 servings
Exchange, 1 serving: 1¾ fruit
Calories, 1 serving: 75
Carbohydrates, 1 serving: 19

Cranberry-Apple Fizz

1½ c.	cranberry-juice cocktail	375 mL
3 c.	apple juice	750 mL
16-oz. bottle	seltzer water	500-mL bottle
14 slices	lemon	14 slices

Combine cranberry-juice cocktail and apple juice in pitcher or glass container. Chill thoroughly. Just before serving, add seltzer water. Pour into ice-filled glass; then garnish with lemon slice.

Yield: 14 servings
Exchange, 1 serving: 1 fruit
Calories, 1 serving: 43
Carbohydrates, 1 serving: 10

Fresh Homemade Lemonade

¾ c.	freshly squeezed lemon juice	190 mL
4¾ c.	cold water	1190 mL
5 env.	aspartame low-calorie sweetener	5 env.

Combine juice, water, and sweetener in a large glass jar or pitcher. Stir to blend. Pour over chipped ice or cubes in tall glasses.

Yield: 4 servings
Exchange, 1 serving: ½ fruit
Calories, 1 serving: 18
Carbohydrates, 1 serving: 4

Chocolate Malted Milk

1 c.	cold skim milk	250 mL
2 T.	chocolate malted-milk powder	30 mL
2 T.	low-calorie chocolate syrup	30 mL
⅔ c.	vanilla ice cream	180 mL

Combine milk, malted-milk powder, and chocolate syrup. Beat until frothy. Add ice cream and beat until well blended. Pour into two glasses.

Yield: 2 servings
Exchange, 1 serving: 1 nonfat milk, ¾ bread
Calories, 1 serving: 134
Carbohydrates, 1 serving: 24

Citrus-Rum Cup

1	orange	1
1	lemon	1
1	lime	1
1 c.	shaved ice	250 mL
⅓ c.	orange juice	90 mL
2 t.	granulated sugar replacement	10 mL
1 t.	rum flavoring	5 mL
½ c.	cold water	125 mL

Cut orange, lemon, and lime. Squeeze juice from fruit; then pour over shaved ice in blender container. Remove membrane from fruit shells, and then cut fruit shells into thin strips. Set aside for garnish. Add remaining ingredients to blender. Blend thoroughly. Pour into two well-chilled glasses. Decorate with reserved fruit-shell strips.

Yield: 2 servings
Exchange, 1 serving: 1¾ fruit
Calories, 1 serving: 69
Carbohydrates, 1 serving: 18

Tex-Mex Chocolate

1 c.	hot skim milk	250 mL
1 oz.	German's Sweet Chocolate, melted	28 g
1 T.	instant coffee	15 mL
1½ T.	granulated sugar replacement	22 mL
¼ t.	vanilla extract	1 mL
¼ t.	cinnamon	1 mL
dash	salt	dash
1 c.	cold skim milk	250 mL

Pour the hot milk, melted chocolate, instant coffee, and sugar replacement in a blender. Blend until thoroughly mixed. Add remaining ingredients. Pour over ice cubes in chilled glasses.

Yield: 4 servings
Exchange, 1 serving: ¾ low-fat milk
Calories, 1 serving: 76
Carbohydrates, 1 serving: 8

Pineapple-Strawberry Drink

2 c.	pineapple juice	500 mL
2 c.	strawberry juice	500 mL

Combine ingredients and chill.

Yield: 4 c. (1000 mL) or 8 servings
Exchange, 1 serving: 1½ fruit
Calories, 1 serving: 58
Carbohydrates, 1 serving: 14

Special Fizz

1 c.	fresh pineapple cubes	250 mL
1	egg	1
2 t.	lemon juice	10 mL
2 env.	aspartame low-calorie sweetener	2 env.
1 t.	rum flavoring	5 mL
⅓ c.	shaved ice	90 mL

Combine all ingredients in blender. Blend thoroughly. Pour into chilled glass.

Yield: 1 serving
Exchange: 2 fruit, 1 medium-fat meat
Calories: 160
Carbohydrates: 21

Strawberry Cocktail

1 c.	orange juice	250 mL
1 c.	fresh strawberries	250 mL
1 T.	granulated sugar replacement	15 mL
1 c.	shaved or crushed ice	250 mL

Combine ingredients in blender. Cover and blend at low speed until ice is melted. Serve immediately in chilled glasses.

Yield: 3 servings
Exchange, 1 serving: 1½ fruit
Calories, 1 serving: 58
Carbohydrates, 1 serving: 16

Apricot Bounce

32-oz. can	apricots, in their own juice	912-g can
6-oz. can	frozen orange juice	170-g can
1 c.	water	250 mL
3 c.	crushed ice	750 mL
6-oz. can	frozen lemonade	170-g can

Pour apricots and their juice in blender. Cover and blend thoroughly to a purée. Add the frozen orange juice and ½ c. (125 mL) of the water and 1 c. (250 mL) of the crushed ice. Blend thoroughly. Pour into large pitcher. Pour the frozen lemonade into blender with the remaining ½ c. (125 mL) of water. Blend thoroughly. Add to apricot mixture in pitcher. Stir to mix. Next, add the remaining 2 c. (500 mL) of crushed ice. Pour over ice cubes in tall glasses.

Yield: 12 servings
Exchange, 1 serving: 3½ fruit
Calories, 1 serving: 105
Carbohydrates, 1 serving: 35

Sunshine Tea

6-oz. can	frozen pineapple-orange juice	177-g can
¼ c.	unsweetened instant tea	60 mL
1 T.	granulated brown-sugar replacement	15 mL
½ t.	cinnamon	2 mL
¼ t.	nutmeg	1 mL
5 c.	water	1250 mL

Combine ingredients in saucepan. While stirring, heat thoroughly. Pour into mugs. You can also make this tea ahead of time; then store it and reheat it as needed.

Yield: 6 servings
Exchange, 1 serving: 1½ fruit
Calories, 1 serving: 60
Carbohydrates, 1 serving: 14

Peach Ice-Cream Cooler

1	peach, peeled and sliced	1
½ c.	skim milk	125 mL
2 drops	almond extract	2 drops
⅓ c.	vanilla ice cream	90 mL

Combine peach slices, skim milk, and almond extract in blender. Blend until smooth. Add ice cream. Blend on low until slightly blended. Pour into chilled glasses immediately.

Yield: 2 servings
Exchange, 1 serving: ½ fruit, ½ starch/bread
Calories, 1 serving: 75
Carbohydrates, 1 serving: 15

Quick Pick-Up

½ c.	orange juice	125 mL
1	egg	1
3	ice cubes	3

Combine orange juice and egg in blender. Cover and blend slightly. Add ice cubes. Blend on low speed for 2 minutes (ice cubes will not be completely crushed). Pour into glass.

Yield: 1 serving
Exchange: 1 fruit, 1 medium-fat meat
Calories: 120
Carbohydrates: 9

Hot Cider

1 qt.	apple cider	1 L
7 whole	cloves	7 whole
2 in.	cinnamon stick	5 cm

Combine ingredients in saucepan. Bring just to boiling point; then reduce heat and simmer 3 minutes. Strain and serve.

Yield: 6 servings
Exchange, 1 serving: 2 fruit
Calories, 1 serving: 80
Carbohydrates, 1 serving: 20

Heavenly Melon Drink

¼	cantaloupe	¼
1 t.	vanilla extract	5 mL
1 env.	aspartame low-calorie sweetener	1 env.
1 c.	skim milk	250 mL

Peel rind from cantaloupe, and cut into chunks. Combine cantaloupe, vanilla, and sweetener in blender. Blend until melon is puréed. Add milk and continue blending on low speed to mix. Pour into chilled glasses.

Yield: 2 servings
Exchange, 1 serving: ½ nonfat milk, ½ fruit
Calories, 1 serving: 60
Carbohydrates, 1 serving: 11

Pink Pleasure

1 c.	low-calorie cranberry-juice cocktail	250 mL
¼ c.	orange juice	60 mL
1 c.	vanilla ice milk	250 mL

Combine ingredients in blender. Cover and blend until smooth. Serve immediately

Yield: 3 servings
Exchange, 1 serving: 1 fruit, ½ low-fat milk
Calories, 1 serving: 103
Carbohydrates, 1 serving: 17

Cider Zip

1 c.	apple cider	250 mL
¼ c.	strained orange juice	60 mL
½ t.	granulated sugar replacement	2 mL
1 t.	lemon juice	5 mL

Combine all ingredients in saucepan. Heat thoroughly.

Yield: 1 serving
Exchange: 3⅓ fruit
Calories: 146
Carbohydrates: 36

Pineapple Splash

1 c.	diced fresh pineapple	250 mL
3	oranges, peeled and cut into pieces	3
½ c.	water	125 mL
2 t.	wintergreen flavoring	10 mL
1 c.	shaved or crushed ice	250 mL

Combine pineapple, oranges, and water in blender. Cover and blend into a liquid. Add flavoring and shaved ice. Blend on low speed until ice is completely melted.

Yield: 4 servings
Exchange, 1 serving: 1¾ fruit
Calories, 1 serving: 69
Carbohydrates, 1 serving: 17

Tropical Magic Drink

2	limes	2
2	oranges	2
1	papaya	1
1	mango	1
1	banana	1
1 qt.	pineapple juice	1 L
2 c.	water	500 mL
2	vanilla beans, split lengthwise	2
3 T.	granulated sugar replacement	45 mL

Peel, seed, and chop fruits. Put small amounts of fruit in food processor or blender, and then process to coarse purée. Combine fruit purée, pineapple juice, water, and vanilla beans in saucepan. While stirring, cook over low heat until very warm. Strain juices into another saucepan or pitcher. Add sugar replacement to juices; then stir to dissolve. Serve immediately. You can also store this drink in the refrigerator and serve it cold.

Yield: 8 servings
Exchange, 1 serving: 3 fruit
Calories, 1 serving: 112
Carbohydrates, 1 serving: 28

Mulled Grape Juice

1 qt.	grape juice	1 L
1 c.	water	250 mL
4 in.	cinnamon stick	10 cm
10 whole	cloves	10 whole
⅓ c.	lemon juice	90 mL

Combine grape juice, water, cinnamon stick, and cloves in saucepan. Bring to boil; then reduce heat and simmer very low for 12 minutes. Remove cinnamon stick and cloves. Add lemon juice. Stir and serve.

Yield: 8 servings
Exchange, 1 serving: 2 fruit
Calories, 1 serving: 82
Carbohydrates, 1 serving: 21

Hot Cranberry Cocktail

32-oz. can	cranberry-juice cocktail	896-g can
2 T.	granulated brown-sugar replacement	30 mL
4 whole	cloves	4 whole
2 sticks	cinnamon	2 sticks

Combine ingredients in saucepan. Stir and cook over low heat until hot. Pour into mugs.

Yield: 6 servings
Exchange, 1 serving: 1½ fruit
Calories, 1 serving: 55
Carbohydrates, 1 serving: 14

Hot and Creamy Eggnog

2 c.	2% low-fat milk	500 mL
1	egg, separated	1
2 env.	aspartame low-calorie sweetener	2 env.

Heat the milk over low heat until warm. Whisk or beat the egg white until frothy. Beat the egg yolk into the warmed milk. Add sweetener. Then fold in egg white. Serve immediately.

Yield: 2 servings
Exchange, 1 serving: 1 low-fat milk, ½ medium-fat meat
Calories, 1 serving: 165
Carbohydrates, 1 serving: 13

Watermelon Fizz

1 c.	watermelon pieces (seeds removed)	250 mL
1 env.	aspartame low-calorie sweetener	1 env.
12-oz. bottle	white wine cooler	355-mL bottle

Combine watermelon and sweetener in blender. Cover and blend to purée watermelon. Pour into a pitcher. Add wine cooler and stir to mix. Pour over ice cubes in chilled glasses.

Yield: 2 servings
Exchange, 1 serving: ½ fruit, 1 starch/bread, 1 fat
Calories, 1 serving: 147
Carbohydrate, 1 serving: 21

Blueberry Bounce

1 c.	blueberries	250 mL
½ c.	skim milk	125 mL
2 t.	granulated sugar replacement	10 mL
1 t.	lemon juice	5 mL
2 c.	seltzer water	500 mL

Combine blueberries, skim milk, sugar replacement, and lemon juice in blender. Cover and blend thoroughly. Add seltzer water, and stir mixture with long spoon. Pour over crushed ice in tall glasses.

Yield: 3 servings
Exchange, 1 serving: 1 fruit
Calories, 1 serving: 43
Carbohydrates, 1 serving: 8

Hot Spiced Tomato Juice

6-oz. can	tomato juice	170-mL
½ t.	lemon juice	2 mL
dash each	Worcestershire sauce, nutmeg, salt	dash each

Combine ingredients in a small saucepan or cup. Stir to blend. Heat just to boiling over stove burner or in microwave oven.

Yield: 1 serving
Exchange: 1 fruit
Calories: 37
Carbohydrates: 9

Salads & Vegetables

Tomato-Potato Salad

1 pkg.	au gratin potatoes	1 pkg.
3 c.	water	750 mL
¾ c.	water	190 mL
1 pkg.	cheese-sauce mix	1 pkg.
⅓ c.	low-calorie salad dressing	90 mL
1 t.	prepared yellow mustard	5 mL
2	eggs, hard-cooked	2
½ c.	coarsely chopped celery	125 mL
8	tomatoes	8

Combine dry potato slices and the 3 c. (750 mL) water in a medium-sized saucepan. Heat to boiling; then reduce heat and simmer, covered, for 15 to 20 minutes or until potatoes are just fork-tender. Rinse immediately with cold water. Drain well; then cover and chill thoroughly. In a small saucepan, combine the ¾ c. (190 mL) water and the package of dry cheese-sauce mix. While stirring, cook over medium heat until mixture boils and thickens. Remove from heat and chill. To serve: Combine chilled cheese sauce, salad dressing, and mustard. Stir to blend thoroughly. Peel hard-cooked eggs and slice into chilled potatoes. Add celery to potatoes and fold in gently. Then fold in salad-dressing mixture. With the stem side down, cut tomatoes into eight wedges. Do not cut through the base of the tomato. Spread wedges apart slightly. Fill with salad. You can also make the filling beforehand and stuff the tomatoes when needed.

Yield: 8 servings
Exchange, 1 serving: 1 starch/bread, 1 fat
Calories, 1 serving: 118
Carbohydrates, 1 serving: 18

Relish Salad

2 env.	dietetic lemon-flavor gelatin	2 env.
1 t.	salt	5 mL
2 c.	boiling water	500 mL
2 t.	cider vinegar	10 mL
¾ c.	sliced celery	190 mL
¼ c.	chopped green pepper	60 mL
2 T.	sweet pickle relish	30 mL
1 T.	finely chopped onion	15 mL
6 leaves	lettuce	6 leaves

Dissolve gelatin and salt in the boiling water. Stir in vinegar. Chill until slightly thickened. Combine remaining ingredients in a bowl. Fold to mix. Fold vegetables into slightly thickened gelatin. Pour into six individual moulds. Chill until firm. Then unmould each serving onto a crisp lettuce leaf.

Yield: 6 servings
Exchange, 1 serving: negligible
Calories, 1 serving: 9
Carbohydrates, 1 serving: 1

Sprout and Shrimp Salad

1-lb. can	bean sprouts	489-g can
1 T.	olive oil	15 mL
½ c.	finely chopped onion	125 mL
6-oz. pkg.	small cooked shrimp	170-g pkg.
1½ T.	soy sauce	22 mL
dash	black pepper	dash

Drain bean sprouts; then rinse thoroughly and drain again. Heat oil in skillet; then add onion. Sauté until lightly browned. Next, add bean sprouts, shrimp, soy sauce, and pepper. Toss to mix well. Heat thoroughly. Serve hot.

Yield: 2 servings
Exchange, 1 serving: ½ vegetable, 1 lean meat
Calories, 1 serving: 72
Carbohydrates, 1 serving: 3

Hot Slaw

1 T.	low-calorie margarine	15 mL
2 c.	shredded cabbage	500 mL
¼ c.	water	60 mL
½ t.	salt	2 mL
1 T.	white vinegar	15 mL
2 t.	granulated sugar replacement	10 mL
½ t.	Dijon-style mustard	2 mL
2 T.	low-calorie sour cream	30 mL
2 T.	low-calorie salad dressing	30 mL

Melt margarine in a medium-sized saucepan; then add cabbage and stir to completely coat. Add water and salt. Stir slightly. Cover and simmer for 10 minutes. Drain thoroughly. Return saucepan to top of burner. Stir in vinegar, sugar replacement, and mustard. Cover and simmer over very low heat for 1 minute. Combine sour cream and salad dressing in a bowl, and then fold this mixture into cabbage. Serve hot.

Yield: 2 servings
Exchange, 1 serving: 2 vegetable, 1 fat
Calories, 1 serving: 102
Carbohydrates, 1 serving: 9

Pineapple-Yogurt Salad

3 c.	shredded iceberg lettuce	750 mL
1½ c.	chopped endive	375 mL
¼ c.	low-calorie pineapple yogurt	60 mL
1 t.	salt	5 mL
½ t.	wintergreen flavoring	2 mL

Mix lettuce and endive together in a large bowl. In a separate bowl, combine yogurt, salt, and wintergreen flavoring; then stir to blend. Add small amounts of yogurt mixture to lettuce and endive; then toss until thoroughly blended. Chill thoroughly.

Yield: 3 servings
Exchange, 1 serving: 1 fruit
Calories, 1 serving: 38
Carbohydrates, 1 serving: 9

Spinach and Bacon Salad

1 lb.	spinach	500 g
4 slices	bacon, crisply fried	4 slices
¼ c.	low-calorie Italian dressing	60 mL

Rinse and drain spinach; then tear into bite-sized pieces. Crumble bacon into small pieces. Combine spinach, bacon, and dressing in a salad bowl. Toss lightly to mix. This salad is one of my favorites.

Yield: 4 servings
Exchange, 1 serving: 1 vegetable, 1 fat
Calories, 1 serving: 67
Carbohydrates, 1 serving: 3

Four-Bean Salad

1-lb. can	green beans	489-g can
1-lb. can	yellow wax beans	489-g can
1-lb. can	red kidney beans	489-g can
1-lb. can	green lima beans	489-g can
1	onion, chopped	1
1 c.	chopped celery	250 mL
½ c.	chopped green pepper	125 mL
¾ c.	sunflower oil	190 mL
½ c.	white vinegar	125 mL
½ c.	granulated sugar replacement	125 mL
2 t.	salt	10 mL
½ t.	black pepper	2 mL

Drain and rinse all of the beans; then drain them again. Mix the beans together in a large bowl. Fold in onion, celery, and green pepper. Combine remaining ingredients in a blender. Blend on high speed for 1 minute. Pour this vinegar-oil mixture over the beans, and toss to completely coat the beans. Turn into a large covered glass bowl; then refrigerate at least 24 hours. Serve the salad with a slotted spoon. It's a good idea to have this simple recipe always prepared and stored in your refrigerator.

Yield: 12 servings
Exchange, 1 serving: 1 starch/bread, ½ vegetable, 1 fat
Calories, 1 serving: 126
Carbohydrates, 1 serving: 15

Herb Cottage-Cheese Salad

1 lb.	low-calorie cottage cheese	500 g
½ c.	low-calorie sour cream	125 mL
½ c.	peeled and chopped cucumber	125 mL
⅓ c.	chopped green pepper	90 mL
1 T.	chopped chives	15 mL
pinch each	dill seed, tarragon, summer savory	pinch each
8 leaves	iceberg lettuce	8 leaves

Combine cottage cheese, sour cream, cucumber, green pepper, and herbs in a bowl. Stir to mix. Cover and refrigerate for at least 2 hours. Arrange lettuce leaves on eight plates. Mound cottage-cheese salad in middle of each leaf.

Yield: 8 servings
Exchange, 1 serving: 1 low-fat milk, ½ fat
Calories, 1 serving: 145
Carbohydrates, 1 serving: 12

Parmesan Asparagus

1 T.	butter	15 mL
1 T.	all-purpose flour	15 mL
¼ c.	chicken broth or water	60 mL
¼ c.	skim milk	60 mL
2 T.	shredded Cheddar cheese	30 mL
3 T.	grated Parmesan cheese	45 mL
¼ t.	salt	1 mL
¼ t.	black pepper	1 mL
1 lb.	asparagus, cooked and hot	500 g

Melt butter in small skillet. Stir in flour to make a paste. Gradually add chicken broth and milk. While stirring, cook until mixture thickens. Stir in Cheddar cheese, 2 T. (30 mL) of the Parmesan cheese, and the salt and pepper. Stir until cheeses melt. Place cooked asparagus on oven-proof baking plate or platter. Pour cheese sauce over asparagus. Sprinkle with the remaining 1 T. (15 mL) of Parmesan cheese. Place under broiler in oven, and broil until surface is slightly browned.

Yield: 4 servings
Exchange, 1 serving: 1 vegetable, 1 fat
Calories, 1 serving: 62
Carbohydrates, 1 serving: 6

Apple and Cranberry Relish

6	apples, cored	6
1	orange, peeled and seeded	1
1 lb.	cranberries	498 g
6 env.	aspartame low-calorie sweetener	6 env.

Cut apples and orange into sections. Grind fruit sections and cranberries through the large hole on a food grinder. Stir in sweetener. Place in a covered glass jar or bowl. Refrigerate.

Yield: 12 servings
Exchange, 1 serving: 1 fruit
Calories, 1 serving: 45
Carbohydrates, 1 serving: 11

Applesauce Salad

3 c.	unsweetened applesauce	750 mL
1 pkg.	dietetic raspberry-flavor gelatin	1 pkg.
1 c.	diet lemon-lime soda	250 mL

Heat applesauce in large saucepan. When hot, add gelatin. Stir until gelatin is dissolved. Remove from heat; allow to cool slightly. Stir in lemon-lime soda. Chill to set firm.

Yield: 8 servings
Exchange, 1 serving: 1 fruit
Calories, 1 serving: 42
Carbohydrates, 1 serving: 11

Green Beans Amandine

1-lb. can	green beans, French-style	489-g can
2 T.	low-calorie margarine	30 mL
¼ c.	slivered almonds	60 mL
	salt and pepper to taste	

Drain beans. Melt margarine in skillet. Add almonds and sauté until lightly browned. Add beans and warm thoroughly. Next, add salt and pepper to taste.

Yield: 6 servings
Exchange, 1 serving: 1 vegetable, ½ fat
Calories, 1 serving: 55
Carbohydrates, 1 serving: 4

Cheesy Zucchini

1 lb.	zucchini	500 g
2 T.	low-calorie margarine	30 mL
1	white onion, chopped	1
1 clove	garlic, minced	1
1 lb.	tomatoes	500 g
2 T.	snipped fresh parsley	30 mL
¾ c.	shredded Cheddar cheese	190 mL
	black pepper	

Wash and cut zucchini into 2-in. (5-cm) slices. Melt margarine in a skillet. Sauté onion and garlic in the margarine until transparent. Add zucchini and sauté for 5 minutes or until zucchini is almost tender. Peel and chop tomatoes. Add parsley to tomatoes and toss to incorporate. In the bottom of a lightly greased baking dish, place a layer of tomatoes; then add a layer of zucchini. Sprinkle with ½ of the shredded Cheddar cheese and a small amount of black pepper. Finish with a layer of tomatoes, a layer of zucchini, and a layer of cheese. Bake at 350 °F (175 °C) for 40 to 45 minutes.

Yield: 6 servings
Exchange, 1 serving: 1 vegetable, 1 fat
Calories, 1 serving: 68
Carbohydrates, 1 serving: 4

Stuffed Mushrooms

1 lb.	fresh mushrooms	500 g
1 c.	low-calorie cottage cheese	250 mL
2 T.	finely chopped chives	30 mL
½ t.	Worcestershire sauce	2 mL
½ t.	Dijon-style mustard	2 mL

Clean mushrooms, removing stems. Set caps aside. Chop stems very fine. Combine chopped stems and remaining ingredients in a bowl. Stir to blend. Then fill the mushroom caps with the cottage-cheese mixture. These Stuffed Mushrooms make delicious appetizers.

Yield: 4 servings
Exchange, 1 serving: ½ vegetable, ½ nonfat milk
Calories, 1 serving: 51
Carbohydrates, 1 serving: 2

Brussels Sprouts with Butter Crumbs

1 lb.	Brussels Sprouts, rinsed and trimmed	500 g
3 T.	low-calorie margarine	45 mL
⅓ c.	dry bread crumbs	90 mL
1 env.	natural butter-flavored mix	1 env.
1 T.	lemon juice	15 mL
	freshly ground black pepper	

Cook Brussels Sprouts in boiling water for about 15 minutes or until tender. Drain and transfer to heated baking dish. Keep warm. Melt margarine in small skillet; then add bread crumbs and sauté until golden brown. Sprinkle bread crumbs with butter mix. Toss to completely coat. Stir in lemon juice. Pour over Brussels Sprouts. Sprinkle with black pepper.

Yield: 4 servings
Exchange, 1 serving: 1 vegetable, 1 fat, ½ starch/bread
Calories, 1 serving: 92
Carbohydrates, 1 serving: 11

Sweet Spinach

1 lb.	fresh spinach, rinsed	500 g
¼ c.	white raisins (sultanas)	60 mL
2 T.	granulated sugar replacement	30 mL

Cook spinach in a saucepan of boiling salted water until tender. Drain and rinse with cold water until spinach is cool. Squeeze spinach in both hands to remove moisture. Bring 2 c. (500 mL) of water to a boil, and then add white raisins. Reduce heat and simmer for 3 minutes or until raisins are plumbed. Drain thoroughly. Heat a skillet over medium heat. When a drop of water sizzles on the surface, add spinach and raisins. Quickly toss spinach to heat thoroughly. Then transfer to heated bowl. Sprinkle with sugar replacement. Toss lightly, and serve immediately.

Yield: 3 servings
Exchange, 1 serving: ½ vegetable, ½ fruit
Calories, 1 serving: 47
Carbohydrates, 1 serving: 11

Eggplant, Italian-Style

2 T.	olive oil	30 mL
1	eggplant, coarsely chopped	1
½ c.	thickly sliced celery	125 mL
1	onion, coarsely chopped	1
1	green pepper, sliced	1
2 c.	coarsely chopped tomatoes	500 mL
¼ c.	red wine vinegar	60 mL
1 t.	oregano	5 mL
¼ t.	fennel seed	1 mL
	salt and pepper to taste	

Heat oil in skillet. Add eggplant, celery, and onion. Cook over medium heat until onion is transparent. Add remaining ingredients. Cover and simmer for 20 to 25 minutes. Serve hot, or chill in covered glass bowl.

Yield: 6 servings
Exchange, 1 serving: 1 vegetable, 1 fat
Calories, 1 serving: 67
Carbohydrates, 1 serving: 6

Leeks and Mushrooms

1 lb.	small mushrooms	500 g
6	leeks	6
½	red pepper	½
2 T.	low-calorie margarine	30 mL
	salt and pepper to taste	

Clean mushrooms and remove stems. Thinly slice the white part of the leeks. Slice the red pepper in thin strips. Melt the margarine in a saucepan over low heat. Add vegetables, salt, and pepper. Cover tightly. Allow to cook over low heat for 2 minutes. Remove lid and toss vegetables. Replace lid on saucepan and cook for 2 more minutes. Remove lid and cook over high heat to evaporate any liquid. Transfer to heated plate or chafing dish.

Yield: 3 servings
Exchange, 1 serving: ½ vegetable, 1 fat
Calories, 1 serving: 55
Carbohydrates, 1 serving: 3

Sautéed Cherry Tomatoes

2 t.	olive oil	10 mL
1 clove	garlic, sliced	1 clove
1 c.	cherry tomatoes, rinsed	250 mL
dash each	salt, pepper, basil	dash each

Heat oil in small skillet. Add garlic and cherry tomatoes. Heat by tilting the pan so that the tomatoes roll. Cherry tomatoes cook and burst quickly. Do not overcook. Just as the tomatoes are showing signs of softening, sprinkle with salt, pepper, and basil. Serve immediately. (If you are making a larger quantity than the recipe calls for, cook in a large heavy pan. Do not crowd the tomatoes or prevent them from rolling.)

Yield: 1 serving
Exchange: 1 vegetable, 2 fat
Calories: 103
Carbohydrates: 6

Stir-Fried Vegetables

2 T.	olive oil	30 mL
1 sm. piece	ginger, grated	1 sm. piece
½ c.	chopped onion	125 mL
1	green pepper, cut in strips	1
1	red pepper, cut in strips	1
½ c.	sliced celery	125 mL
½ c.	sliced carrots	125 mL
1 c.	broccoli flowerets	250 mL
1 c.	sliced mushrooms	250 mL
1 T.	soy sauce	15 m

Heat the olive oil in a wok. Add grated ginger and fry for 1 minute. Remove ginger from wok. Add onion, green and red peppers, celery, and carrots. Fry for 3 minutes, tossing vegetables as they fry. Add broccoli and mushrooms. Toss vegetables. Add small amount of water. Cover and allow to simmer for 2 to 3 minutes. Next, add soy sauce. Fry without cover for 1 minute. Serve in wok, or transfer to heated plate or dish.

Yield: 6 servings
Exchange, 1 serving: 1 vegetable, 1 fat
Calories, 1 serving: 65
Carbohydrates, 1 serving: 6

Soups

Cream of Onion Soup

2 T.	low-calorie margarine	30 mL
6	onions, thinly sliced	6
1 T.	all-purpose flour	15 mL
1 qt.	skim milk	1 L
1 c.	evaporated skim milk	250 mL
1 env.	natural butter-flavored mix	1 env.
4	egg yolks, slightly beaten	4
	salt and pepper to taste	

Melt margarine in a saucepan; then add onions. While stirring, cook over low heat until onions begin to soften. Cover and simmer on low heat for 30 minutes. Do not allow onions to burn. Sprinkle flour over onions and stir until liquid in saucepan is smooth. Heat skim milk in top of double boiler. Add onion mixture and cook over simmering water for 50 minutes. Pour mixture into a blender, and blend until smooth. Return mixture to top of double boiler. Combine evaporated milk, butter-flavored mix, and egg yolks; then gradually add to milk-onion mixture. Salt and pepper to taste. Cook over simmering water until hot. If mixture should curdle, beat with an electric mixer.

Yield: 8 servings
Exchange, 1 serving: 1 low-fat milk
Calories, 1 serving: 110
Carbohydrates, 1 serving: 11

Onion Soup

4	onions, thinly sliced	4
2 T.	low-calorie margarine	30 mL
2 (10½ oz.) cans	condensed beef broth	2 (310 g) cans
1 t.	Worcestershire sauce	5 mL
	salt and pepper to taste	
6 slices	French bread	6 slices
6 t.	grated Parmesan cheese	30 mL

Sauté onions in the margarine over low heat until they are golden brown. Add beef broth, Worcestershire sauce, salt, and pepper. Cover and simmer for 25 to 30 minutes. Place a slice of bread in six bowls. Pour the soup over the top of the bread. Sprinkle each bowl of soup with 1 t. (5 mL) of Parmesan cheese.

Yield: 6 servings
Exchange, 1 serving: 1 starch/bread, ¾ lean meat
Calories, 1 serving: 108
Carbohydrates, 1 serving: 17

Borscht

16-oz. jar	sweet-sour cabbage, drained	488-g jar
16-oz. can	shoestring beets	488-g can
10-oz. can	onion soup	289-g can
10-oz. can	condensed beef broth	310-g can
1 c.	water	250 mL
2 t.	freshly snipped parsley	10 mL
1 T.	lemon juice	30 mL
8 T.	low-calorie sour cream	120 mL

Combine the drained sweet-sour cabbage, beets with their liquid, onion soup, beef broth, water, parsley, and lemon juice in a saucepan. Bring to a boil; then reduce heat and simmer for 10 minutes. Spoon 1 T. (15 mL) of sour cream into eight soup bowls. Ladle soup over sour cream. Serve immediately.

Yield: 8 servings
Exchange, 1 serving: 1 vegetable, ⅓ fat
Calories, 1 serving: 40
Carbohydrates, 1 serving: 6

Orange-Beef Soup

2	navel oranges	2
1 T.	low-calorie margarine	15 mL
2 (10 ½ oz.) cans	condensed beef broth	2 (310 g) cans
1 c.	water	250 mL
½ c.	orange juice	125 mL
3 whole	cloves	3 whole
1 T.	granulated sugar replacement	15 mL

With a vegetable peeler, cut six thin strips from the outer zest of the orange. Set aside. Cut all the remaining peel, including the white membrane, from the orange. Working over a pan, separate the orange into sections. Remove the thin membrane from each section. Sauté orange sections in the low-calorie margarine for 3 minutes. Add beef broth, water, orange juice, and cloves. Bring to a boil, reduce heat, and simmer for 10 minutes. Remove cloves. Stir in sugar replacement. Place one reserved orange-zest strip in six individual bowls. Then pour in the soup.

Yield: 6 servings
Exchange, 1 serving: 1 fruit, ¾ fat
Calories, 1 serving: 64
Carbohydrates, 1 serving: 11

Vegetable Soup with Basil

1 c.	water	250 mL
2 t.	sweet basil	10 mL
2 cloves	garlic, sliced	2 cloves
½	bay leaf	½
10¾-oz. can	vegetable soup	300-g can
½ c.	broken vermicelli noodles	125 mL

Combine water, basil, garlic, and bay leaf in a saucepan. Bring to a boil, reduce heat, and simmer for 5 minutes. Strain liquid. To the strained liquid, add vegetable soup and vermicelli noodles. While stirring, cook over low heat until noodles are tender.

Yield: 3 servings
Exchange, 1 serving: 1 starch/bread, ⅓ fat
Calories, 1 serving: 91
Carbohydrates, 1 serving: 17

Fast, Fresh Creamed Tomato Soup

2 c.	peeled and diced tomatoes	500 mL
2 T.	low-calorie margarine	30 mL
2 T.	all-purpose flour	30 mL
1 t.	salt	5 mL
	pepper to taste	
¼ t.	baking soda	1 mL
1 c.	skim milk	250 mL
½ c.	condensed chicken broth	125 mL

Combine tomatoes, margarine, flour, salt, and pepper in a blender. Blend on HIGH until puréed. Pour into a saucepan. While stirring, cook until boiling. Reduce heat and simmer for 3 minutes. Stir in baking soda. Then gradually add milk and chicken broth. Heat thoroughly. Pour into six soup bowls.

Yield: 6 servings
Exchange, 1 serving: ⅓ low-fat milk, ⅓ vegetable
Calories, 1 serving: 47
Carbohydrates, 1 serving: 5

Easy Greek Lemon Soup

2 (10 ½ oz.) cans	condensed chicken broth	2 (310 g) cans
1½ c.	water	375 mL
4	eggs	4
¼ c.	lemon juice	60 mL
1 whole	lemon, thinly sliced	1 whole

Combine chicken broth and water in a saucepan. Heat to boiling, and then reduce heat to very low. Beat eggs until foamy; then beat in lemon juice. Slowly stir some of the hot chicken broth into the egg mixture, beating constantly. Pour egg mixture into the pan of broth, and cook over very low heat until hot and thickened. Remove from heat. Pour into eight heated soup bowls, and garnish with lemon slices.

Yield: 8 servings
Exchange, 1 serving: ½ medium-fat meat
Calories, 1 serving: 38
Carbohydrates, 1 serving: 2

Dutch Vegetable Soup

3 c.	beef broth	750 mL
½ c.	cooked and shredded lean beef	125 mL
1 c.	cooked lima beans	125 mL
2 c.	peeled and chopped tomatoes	500 mL
2 c.	chopped cabbage	500 mL
1 c.	corn	250 mL
1	turnip, diced	1
1	carrot, diced	1
1	onion, chopped	1
	salt and pepper to taste	
1 t.	all-purpose flour	5 mL
⅓ c.	skim milk	90 mL

Combine beef broth, beef, lima beans, tomatoes, cabbage, corn, turnip, carrot, onion, salt, and pepper in a soup pot. Bring to a light boil; then reduce heat and simmer for about 20 minutes or until carrots and turnips are tender. Combine flour and milk in a bowl or shaker bottle. Blend thoroughly. Pour mixture into soup and stir. Cook for an additional 10 minutes. This is a modern version of an old Dutch soup.

Yield: 6 servings
Exchange, 1 serving: 1 starch/bread, ½ medium-fat meat
Calories, 1 serving: 112
Carbohydrates, 1 serving: 14

Wild Rice and Mushroom Soup

1 c.	condensed beef broth	250 mL
½ c.	thinly sliced mushrooms	125 mL
½ c.	cooked wild rice	125 mL
⅓ c.	water	90 mL
2 T.	finely chopped onion	30 mL

Combine all ingredients in a saucepan. Bring to a boil, reduce heat, and simmer for 5 minutes or until mushrooms are tender.

Yield: 2 servings
Exchange, 1 serving: 1 starch/bread
Calories, 1 serving: 66
Carbohydrates, 1 serving: 13

Bacon-Mushroom Soup

2 slices	bacon	2 slices
10¾-oz. can	cream of mushroom soup	378-g can
½ soup can	water	½ soup can
¼ c.	chopped onion	60 mL
dash	freshly ground black pepper	dash

Fry bacon until crisp; then drain and crumble. Combine bacon, soup, water, and onion in a saucepan. While stirring, cook over medium heat until hot. Pour into two soup bowls. Top with freshly ground black pepper.

Yield: 2 servings
Exchange, 1 serving: ½ starch/bread, 2 fat
Calories, 1 serving: 133
Carbohydrates, 1 serving: 8

Old-Fashioned Barley Soup

1 qt.	beef broth	1 L
⅓ c.	quick-cooking barley	90 mL
1	onion, chopped	1
1	carrot, diced	1
½ c.	sliced celery	125 mL
⅔ c.	sliced mushrooms	180 mL
½ t.	salt	2 mL
dash	black pepper	dash
6 t.	low-calorie sour cream	30 mL

Combine beef broth, barley, onion, carrot, celery, mushrooms, salt, and pepper in a soup pot. Cover and simmer until carrots are tender. Spoon into six individual soup dishes. Then top each dish with 1 t. (5 mL) of sour cream.

Yield: 6 servings
Exchange, 1 serving: ¾ starch/bread
Calories, 1 serving: 45
Carbohydrates, 1 serving: 11

Oxtail and Barley Soup

2⅝-oz. pkg.	oxtail soup mix	71-g pkg.
1 qt.	water	1 L
1 c.	thinly sliced celery	250 mL
½ c.	quick-cooking barley	125 mL
⅓ c.	chopped onion	90 mL

Combine soup mix and water in a saucepan. Stir to dissolve mix. Bring to a boil; then add remaining ingredients. Reduce heat and simmer for 10 to 12 minutes or until barley is tender, stirring occasionally. This is a thick, dark, delicious soup.

Yield: 6 servings
Exchange, 1 serving: 1 starch/bread, ⅓ fat
Calories, 1 serving: 82
Carbohydrates, 1 serving: 13

Pepper Pot

10-oz. can	pea soup	304-g can
10-oz. can	tomato soup	304-g can
10-oz. can	pepper pot soup	304-g can
2½ c.	water	750 mL
¼ lb.	ground beef, cooked	125 g
2	tomatoes, peeled and chopped	2
2 cloves	garlic, minced	2 cloves
½	onion, finely chopped	½
2 t.	cayenne pepper	10 mL

Combine all ingredients in a soup pot or large saucepan. Stir to blend. Bring to a boil; then reduce heat and simmer for 10 minutes.

Yield: 8 servings
Exchange, 1 serving: 1½ starch/bread, ½ medium-fat meat
Calories, 1 serving: 158
Carbohydrates, 1 serving: 21

Cream of Lentil Soup

3-oz. pkg.	lentil soup mix	85-g pkg.
2 c.	water	500 mL
2 c.	skim milk	500 mL
3 T.	finely snipped chives	45 mL
	paprika	

Combine soup mix, water, and milk in a saucepan. Stir to dissolve soup mix. While stirring, cook over low heat until soup is hot. Pour into six warmed soup bowls. Top with chives and a dash of paprika.

Yield: 6 servings
Exchange, 1 serving: ½ starch/bread, ½ skim milk
Calories, 1 serving: 81
Carbohydrates, 1 serving: 11

Special Clam Chowder

1 c.	water	250 mL
1	tomato, peeled and chopped	1
⅓ c.	chopped onion	90 mL
¼ c.	thinly sliced celery	60 mL
2 T.	chopped green pepper	30 mL
10-oz. can	clam chowder	305-g can
	salt and pepper to taste	

Combine water, tomato, onion, celery, and green pepper in a large saucepan. Cover and simmer over medium heat until vegetables are tender. Stir in clam chowder. Add salt and pepper to taste. While stirring, cook over low heat until thoroughly heated.

Yield: 3 servings
Exchange, 1 serving: 2 vegetable
Calories, 1 serving: 53
Carbohydrates, 1 serving: 11

Bean and Pea Soup

10-oz. can	pea soup	304-g can
10-oz. can	bean with bacon soup	304-g can
1½ c.	water	375 mL
⅓ c.	minced onions	90 mL
2	wieners, thinly sliced	2

Combine soups, water, and onions in a saucepan. While stirring, cook over medium heat until hot. Add wieners and cook for an additional 5 minutes.

Yield: 8 servings
Exchange, 1 serving: ¾ starch/bread, ½ high-fat meat
Calories, 1 serving: 94
Carbohydrates, 1 serving: 14

Salmon Tomato Soup

10-oz. can	tomato soup	304-g can
¾ c.	water	190 mL
1 T.	minced onion	15 mL
½ c.	flaked salmon	125 mL
3	lemon slices	3

Combine tomato soup, water, and onion in a saucepan. Heat to boiling; then reduce heat and simmer for 5 minutes. Stir in salmon; then heat for 1 minute. Ladle into three soup bowls. Garnish each bowl with a lemon slice.

Yield: 3 servings
Exchange, 1 serving: 2 vegetables, 1 lean meat
Calories, 1 serving: 105
Carbohydrates, 1 serving: 11

Shrimp Bouillabaisse

6-oz. can	tomato paste	170-g can
4 c.	water	1000 mL
2 whole	cloves	2 whole
2	bay leaves	2
2 t.	salt	10 mL
2 c.	chopped mushrooms	500 mL
½ c.	chopped onion	125 mL
1 clove	garlic, minced	1 clove
¾ t.	curry powder	4 mL
6-oz. pkg.	frozen cooked shrimp	170-g pkg.
½ c.	grated American cheese	125 mL
¼ c.	dry sherry	60 mL
1 T.	all-purpose flour	15 mL

Combine tomato paste, water, cloves, bay leaves, and salt in a large saucepan. Stir to blend. Bring to a boil; then reduce heat, cover, and simmer for 10 minutes. Remove cloves and bay leaves. Add mushrooms, onion, garlic, and curry powder. Simmer until vegetables are tender. Add shrimps and cheese. Stir to blend. Combine sherry and flour in a bowl or cup. Stir to blend. Pour sherry-flour mixture into soup. While stirring, cook until slightly thickened.

Yield: 6 servings
Exchange, 1 serving: ½ medium-fat meat, 1½ vegetables
Calories, 1 serving: 71
Carbohydrates, 1 serving: 8

Tomato Shrimp Bisque

¾ c.	water	190 mL
10-oz. can	tomato soup	304-g can
¼ c.	chopped onion	60 mL
6-oz. pkg.	frozen cooked shrimp, slightly thawed	170-g pkg.

Combine ingredients in a blender in order given. Blend into a purée. Pour into a saucepan. Heat just to boiling; then serve immediately.

Yield: 3 servings
Exchange, 1 serving: 2 vegetable, 1 lean meat
Calories, 1 serving: 102
Carbohydrates, 1 serving: 11

Sandwiches

Salmon Salad

8-oz. can	salmon	240-g can
¼ c.	chopped onion	60 mL
¼ c.	peeled, seeded and chopped cucumber	60 mL
2 T.	chopped parsley	30 mL
½ t.	celery seed	2 mL
2 T.	low-calorie salad dressing	30 mL
1 T.	prepared mustard	15 mL
1 T.	ketchup	15 mL
8	starch/bread exchanges	8
8 slices	tomato	8 slices

Remove skin and bones from salmon. Drain thoroughly and flake. Add onion, cucumber, parsley, celery seed, salad dressing, mustard, and ketchup. Stir to mix. Spread salmon mixture on starch/bread exchanges. Top each sandwich half with a tomato slice. Serve cold or put sandwiches on cookie sheet and place under broiler for 30 seconds. For appetizers, cut each sandwich diagonally in half.

Sandwich Yield: 8 servings
Exchange, 1 serving: 1 starch/bread, ¾ lean meat
Calories, 1 serving: 128
Carbohydrates, 1 serving: 16

Appetizer Yield: 16 servings
Exchange, 1 serving: ½ starch/bread, ½ lean meat
Calories, 1 serving: 64
Carbohydrates, 1 serving: 8

Shrimp Filling

6-oz. pkg.	frozen cooked shrimp, thawed and drained	170-g pkg.
⅓ c.	finely chopped celery	90 mL
⅓ c.	finely chopped bamboo shoots	90 mL
¼ c.	chopped bean sprouts	60 mL
3 T.	low-calorie salad dressing	45 mL

Combine shrimp, celery, bamboo shoots, bean sprouts, and salad dressing in a bowl. (The bamboo shoots add a nutty flavor.) Toss gently to mix.

Sandwich Yield: 4 servings
Exchange, 1 serving: 1 lean meat, ⅓ fat
Calories, 1 serving: 65
Carbohydrates, 1 serving: 2

Appetizer Yield: 8 servings
Exchange, 1 serving: ½ lean meat
Calories, 1 serving: 30
Carbohydrates, 1 serving: 1

Crab Filling

7-oz. can	crab meat	199-g can
⅓ c.	finely chopped celery	90 mL
2 T.	finely chopped onion	30 mL
2 T.	finely grated carrot	30 mL
⅓ c.	low-calorie salad dressing	90 mL
1 t.	Dijon-style mustard	5 mL
	alfalfa sprouts	

Combine crab meat, celery, onion, carrot, salad dressing, and mustard in a bowl. Toss gently to mix. Top with alfalfa sprouts.

Yield: 6 servings
Exchange, 1 serving: ½ lean meat; ½ fat
Calories, 1 serving: 47
Carbohydrates, 1 serving: negligible

Cheesy Eggs

4	eggs, hard-cooked and chopped	4
1 c.	shredded Cheddar cheese	250 mL
3-oz. pkg.	cream cheese, softened	80-g pkg.
2 T.	skim milk	30 mL
¼ t.	salt	1 mL
⅛ t.	black pepper	½ mL

Combine eggs and Cheddar cheese in a bowl. Toss to mix. Combine cream cheese, milk, salt, and pepper in another bowl. Beat to blend. Add to egg-cheese mixture; then fold to mix. This taste good spread on cocktail rye bread.

Yield: 10 servings
Exchange, 1 serving: 1 high-fat meat
Calories, 1 serving: 107
Carbohydrates, 1 serving: 6

Sweet-Sour Chicken

¼ c.	crushed pineapple, in its own juice	60 mL
2 t.	vinegar	10 mL
½ t.	cornstarch	2 mL
1 c.	chopped cooked chicken	250 mL
2 T.	chopped celery	30 mL
1 T.	chopped green onion	15 mL
1 T.	finely chopped almonds	15 mL
1 c.	shredded lettuce	250 mL
2	starch/bread exchanges	2

Combine crushed pineapple, vinegar, and cornstarch in a small saucepan. Stir to dissolve cornstarch. Cook mixture over medium heat until clear and thickened. Cool completely. Combine chicken, celery, green onion, and almonds in a bowl. Add pineapple mixture. Toss to mix. Spread sweet-sour chicken on the starch or bread of your choice; then top with shredded lettuce.

Yield: 2 servings
Exchange, 1 serving: 2½ lean meat, ½ fruit, 1 starch/bread
Calories, 1 serving: 235
Carbohydrates, 1 serving: 22

Chicken Cucumber

1 c.	diced cooked chicken	250 mL
⅓ c.	chopped cucumber	90 mL
¼ c.	low-calorie blue-cheese salad dressing	60 mL
1 c.	shredded lettuce	250 mL

Combine chicken, cucumber, and salad dressing in a bowl. Toss to mix. Fill sandwiches and then top with shredded lettuce. (This filling is excellent in pita pockets.)

Yield: 8 servings
Exchange, 1 serving: 1 lean meat
Calories, 1 serving: 45
Carbohydrates, 1 serving: negligible

Beef Beauties

1 c.	cooked beef (fat removed)	250 mL
½ c.	sliced celery	125 mL
¼	onion	¼
1 t.	Dijon-style mustard	5 mL
4	starch/bread exchanges	4

Combine beef, celery, onion, and mustard in food processor. With its steel blade, process the mixture until the meat is finely shredded. (If you don't have a food processor, finely chop the ingredients.) Pile beef mixture on two starch/bread exchanges. Top each sandwich with another starch/bread exchange. Cut in half. For appetizers, cut four starch/bread exchanges into four squares; then divide beef mixture evenly between the sixteen squares. If desired, top each appetizer with a slice of pimento.

Sandwich Yield: 4 servings
Exchange, 1 serving: 1 starch/bread, 1½ medium-fat meat
Calories, 1 serving: 192
Carbohydrates, 1 serving: 16

Appetizer Yield: 16 servings
Exchange, 1 serving: ½ starch/bread, ¾ medium-fat meat
Calories, 1 serving: 96
Carbohydrates, 1 serving: 8

Turkey and Water Chestnuts

1 c.	chopped cooked turkey	250 mL
2 T.	finely chopped celery	30 mL
2 T.	finely chopped water chestnuts	30 mL
¼ c.	low-calorie salad dressing	60 mL
½ t.	poultry seasoning	2 mL
	salt and pepper to taste	

Combine turkey, celery, water chestnuts, salad dressing, poultry seasoning, salt, and pepper in a bowl. Toss to mix. This is good on rice cakes.

Yield: 5 servings
Exchange, 1 serving: 1 lean meat; ⅓ fat
Calories, 1 serving: 69
Carbohydrates, 1 serving: negligible

French-Toasted Salmon Sandwiches

8-oz. can	salmon	250-g can
3 T.	low-calorie salad dressing	45 mL
2 t.	grated onion	10 mL
½ t.	salt	2 mL
⅛ t.	black pepper	½ mL
8 slices	low-calorie white bread	8 slices
1	egg	1
1 T.	skim milk	15 mL

Drain salmon, reserving liquid. Remove bones, and flake. Add salad dressing, onion, salt, and pepper to salmon; then toss to mix. Spread salmon mixture on four slices of bread; then top each with remaining slices of bread. Combine egg, skim milk, and reserved salmon liquid in a flat bowl. With a whip or fork, beat to blend. Dip sandwiches into the egg mixture, coating both sides. Fry in a skillet sprayed with vegetable oil over medium heat until browned on both sides. Cut in half. Serve hot.

Yield: 8 servings
Exchange, 1 serving: 1 lean meat, ½ starch/bread
Calories, 1 serving: 90
Carbohydrates, 1 serving: 6

Chicken Delight

¼ c.	finely chopped cooked chicken	60 mL
1 T.	finely chopped green pepper	15 mL
1 T.	finely chopped onion	15 mL
¼ t.	poultry seasoning	1 mL

Combine chicken, green pepper, onion, and poultry seasoning in a bowl. With a spoon, stir to make mixture sticky. If needed, add 1 or 2 drops of water.

Yield: 1 serving
Exchange: 1 lean meat
Calories: 60
Carbohydrates: negligible

Ham and Apple Rounds

¼ c.	apple juice	60 mL
½ t.	cornstarch	2 mL
1 c.	chopped ham	250 mL
2	apples, peeled and chopped	2
¼ t.	black pepper	1 mL
⅛ t.	allspice	½ mL
⅛ t.	nutmeg	½ mL

Combine apple juice and cornstarch in a small saucepan. Stir to dissolve cornstarch. Cook over medium heat until mixture is clear and thick. Cool completely. Combine ham, apples, pepper, allspice, and nutmeg in a bowl. Toss to mix. Stir in the cooled apple juice and cornstarch mixture. Chill. I like to use this spread on rice cakes.

Yield: 4 servings
Exchange, 1 serving: 1½ high-fat meat, ¾ fruit
Calories, 1 serving: 203
Carbohydrates, 1 serving: 11

Beef Becquée

1 c.	cooked beef (fat removed)	250 mL
½ c.	chopped celery	125 mL
1 small	onion, chopped	1 small
¼ c.	ketchup	60 mL
2 T.	prepared mustard	30 mL
2 T.	water	30 mL
1 T.	Worcestershire sauce	15 mL
4	starch/bread exchanges	4

Combine beef, celery, and onion in a food processor. With the steel blade, process until beef is shredded. Turn into a saucepan. Add ketchup, mustard, water, and Worcestershire sauce. Heat thoroughly. Pile on starch/bread exchanges. This is great on a hamburger bun.

Yield: 2 servings
Exchange, 1 serving: 2 starch/bread, 3 medium-fat meat
Calories, 1 serving: 384
Carbohydrates, 1 serving: 31

Ham and Cheese Biscuits

6	biscuits, split	6
2 t.	prepared mustard	10 mL
1 t.	horseradish	5 mL
3-oz. pkg.	thinly sliced ham	86-g pkg.
1 c.	shredded Cheddar cheese	250 mL

Spread both top and bottom halves of each biscuit with mustard and horseradish. Divide the ham evenly between the bottom halves of the biscuits. Top the ham with cheese. Place ham and cheese biscuits under the broiler until cheese starts to melt. Cover with the top halves of the biscuits.

Yield: 6 servings
Exchange, 1 serving: 1 starch/bread, 1 high-fat meat
Calories, 1 serving: 196
Carbohydrates, 1 serving: 13

Pile-High Porkies

1 c.	cooked pork (fat removed)	250 mL
⅓ c.	chopped green onion	90 mL
¼ c.	chopped carrot	60 mL
2 T.	Dijon-style mustard	30 mL
2	hamburger rolls, split	2
¼ c.	shredded Cheddar cheese	60 mL

Combine pork, green onion, carrot, and mustard in a food processor. With the steel blade, process until meat is shredded. Under the broiler, toast the bottom half of each roll. Divide pork mixture evenly between the two toasted bottom halves. Sprinkle Cheddar cheese on top of pork mixture. Place sandwich on broiler pan. Place top halves of rolls on broiler pan, with top sides down. Then place under broiler until cheese is melted and insides of top halves of rolls are golden brown.

Yield: 2 servings
Exchange, 1 serving: 3½ high-fat meat, 2 starch/bread
Calories, 1 serving: 508
Carbohydrates, 1 serving: 31

Dilly Beef

¼ lb.	ground beef	125 g
1 t.	dill weed	5 mL
1 t.	ketchup	5 mL
½ t.	prepared mustard	2 mL
	salt and pepper to taste	

Combine beef, dill weed, ketchup, mustard, salt, and pepper in a bowl. With your hands or a spoon, thoroughly blend. Form meat into two patties. Then fry in a skillet or on a grill over hot coals to desired doneness. The dill weed in the beef adds a new taste to an old favorite.

Yield: 2 servings
Exchange, 1 serving: 1¾ medium-fat meat
Calories, 1 serving: 123
Carbohydrates, 1 serving: negligible

Meat, Fish, & Eggs

Lamb Chop with Orange Glaze

½ t.	grated fresh orange peel	2 mL
¼ c.	water	60 mL
¼ c.	orange juice	60 mL
1 T.	cider vinegar	15 mL
1 t.	soy sauce	5 mL
1 t.	granulated brown-sugar replacement	5 mL
dash	black pepper	dash
2	lamb chops	2

Combine orange peel and water in a small saucepan. Bring to a boil, reduce heat, and simmer for 1 minute. Add remaining ingredients, except lamb chops. While stirring, cook until liquid has reduced by one half. Remove from heat. Brush both sides of the lamb chops with orange mixture. Allow to stay at room temperature for 20 minutes. Then brush orange mixture on lamb chops again. Cook lamb chops under the broiler for about 20 minutes or until tender. Turn once. Brush with any remaining glaze during broiling.

Yield: 2 servings
Exchange: 1 high-fat meat
Calories: 100
Carbohydrates: negligible

Crafty Chicken

2 oz.	boned chicken breast	60 g
1 T.	all-purpose flour	15 mL
dash each	salt and pepper	dash each
½ strip	bacon	½ strip

Remove skin from chicken breast. Combine flour, salt, and pepper in a bowl or on a piece of waxed paper. Stir to mix. Roll chicken breast in flour mixture. Place chicken breast in baking dish. Lay the ½ strip of bacon on top of chicken breast. Add ½ in. (1.25 cm) of water. Bake at 350 °F (175 °C) for 30 minutes or until chicken is tender.

Yield: 1 serving
Exchange: 2 lean meat
Calories: 120
Carbohydrates: 5

Great Chicken

4 oz.	boned chicken breast	120 g
1 T.	liquid shortening	15 mL
½	onion, cut in rings	½
3 T.	cider vinegar	45 mL
	salt and pepper to taste	

Remove skin from chicken breast. Heat shortening in skillet, and then brown breast on both sides. Remove from skillet to a small baking dish. Add onion rings to skillet. Fry onion rings until they start to brown slightly. Add cider vinegar to onions in skillet. Cover and reduce heat. Cook for 1 minute. Pour the onion-vinegar mixture over the chicken breast in the baking dish. Season with salt and pepper. Cover and bake at 300 °F (150 °C) for 30 minutes.

Yield: 2 servings
Exchange, 1 serving: 2 lean meat
Calories, 1 serving: 121
Carbohydrates, 1 serving: negligible

Chicken Breast Parmesan

4 oz.	boned chicken breast	120 g
2 T.	all-purpose flour	30 mL
dash each	salt, pepper, oregano	dash each
½ t.	olive oil	2 mL
1 T.	grated Parmesan cheese	15 mL

Remove skin from chicken breast. Place the chicken breast between two pieces of plastic wrap or waxed paper. Using the bottom of a plate, rolling pin, or mallet, flatten chicken breast slightly. Combine flour, salt, pepper, and oregano in a bowl. Stir to mix. Pat flour mixture on both sides of the chicken breast. Heat oil in a nonstick skillet. Add chicken breast and brown both sides. Place chicken breast on hot ovenproof plate or platter. Sprinkle cheese over top of chicken breast. Bake chicken breast in a preheated 400 °F (200 °C) oven for 12 to 15 minutes.

Yield: 2 servings
Exchange, 1 serving: 2 lean meat
Calories, 1 serving: 119
Carbohydrates, 1 serving: 5

Sweet Chicken Breast

4 oz.	boned chicken breast	120 g
1 t.	granulated sugar replacement	5 mL
½ t.	black pepper	2 mL
¼ t.	ground nutmeg	1 mL

Remove skin from chicken breast. Heat ½ c. (125 mL) water to boiling in a small skillet. Add chicken breast. Sprinkle with sugar replacement, pepper, and nutmeg. Cover, reduce heat, and simmer chicken breast for 20 to 25 minutes or until done. (Add small amount of water if needed.)

Yield: 2 servings
Exchange, 1 serving: 2 lean meat
Calories, 1 serving: 108
Carbohydrates, 1 serving: negligible

Paprika and Onion Chicken

½	white onion, chopped	½
1 T.	low-calorie margarine	15 mL
2	chicken thighs	2
2 t.	paprika	10 mL
1 stalk	celery, chopped	1 stalk
1	tomato, chopped	1
	salt and pepper to taste	

Sauté the onions in the margarine until translucent. Add the chicken thighs and brown on both sides. Remove chicken thighs. Add remaining ingredients and small amount of water. Stir to blend. Replace chicken thighs in pan. Cover and simmer for 20 to 35 minutes or until chicken is tender; add small amount of extra water, if needed.

Yield: 2 servings
Exchange: 2 medium-fat meat
Calories: 158
Carbohydrates: 2

Chicken with Ginger

2	chicken thighs	2
¼ c.	cider vinegar	60 mL
3 T.	Worcestershire sauce	45 mL
¼ t.	ground ginger	1 mL

Clean chicken thighs and then remove skin. Combine remaining ingredients in a bowl. Stir to blend. Place thighs in marinade. Cover and refrigerate at least 8 hours or overnight. Place chicken thighs over medium-hot coals on barbecue grill or under oven broiler on middle rack. Turn and baste with marinade every 5 minutes for 15 to 20 minutes. Test for doneness by inserting a fork into the chicken; the meat should move easily.

Yield: 2 servings
Exchange: 1 lean meat
Calories: 49
Carbohydrates: negligible

Chicken Livers and Herbs

1 T.	low-calorie margarine	15 mL
2 T.	chopped red onion	30 mL
½ c.	cleaned chicken livers	125 mL
1 t.	sage	5 mL
½ t.	oregano	2 mL
⅛ t.	crushed fennel	½ mL
	salt and pepper to taste	

Melt the margarine in a skillet. Sauté onions until slightly brown. Add chicken livers, herbs, salt, and pepper. Sauté over high heat until the pink liver juices disappear. Do not overcook. Slide out onto heated plate or heated bed of wilted lettuce. I like to serve this as an appetizer on wilted iceberg lettuce.

Yield: 2 servings
Exchange: 1 medium-fat meat
Calories: 80
Carbohydrates: negligible

Chicken Sauté

4 oz.	skinned and boned chicken breast	120 g
3 T.	whole-wheat flour	45 mL
⅛ t. each	rosemary, thyme, lemon basil	½ mL
	salt and pepper to taste	
2 T.	butter	30 mL

Place the chicken breast between two pieces of plastic wrap or waxed paper. Using the bottom of a plate, rolling pin, or mallet flatten the chicken breast to ¼ in. (8 mm). Combine remaining ingredients, except butter, in a bowl or on a piece of waxed paper. Stir to mix. Dredge the flattened chicken breast in the mixture. Melt the butter in a skillet. Then sauté the chicken breast for 2 to 3 minutes on each side. This is a fast recipe to prepare for a snack. If you want to use it as an appetizer, keep it covered and warm in the oven. Don't let it dry out.

Yield: 2 servings
Exchange: 2 medium-fat meat, ⅓ starch/bread
Calories: 180
Carbohydrates: 7

Chicken Gizzards and Hearts

1 T.	vegetable oil	15 mL
½ c.	cleaned chicken gizzards and hearts	125 mL
½	onion, chopped	½
	salt and pepper to taste	

Heat vegetable oil in skillet. If desired, cut gizzards in half. Add the gizzards and hearts to skillet. Stir and brown evenly. Add onion, salt, and pepper. Reduce heat and cover. Cook for 15 to 20 minutes.

Yield: 2 servings
Exchange: 2 medium-fat meat
Calories: 159
Carbohydrates: 1

Curried Meatballs

Meatballs:

½ lb.	lean ground beef	250 g
2 T.	chopped onion	30 mL
1 small clove	garlic, minced	1 small clove
2 t.	all-purpose flour	10 mL
dash each	allspice, salt, pepper	dash each
2 T.	vegetable oil	30 mL

Curry Sauce:

1 T.	low-calorie margarine	15 mL
½ c.	finely chopped onion	125 mL
½ t.	garlic powder	2 mL
2 t.	curry powder	10 mL
½ c.	water	125 mL
1 cube	chicken bouillon	1 cube
2 t.	tomato paste	10 mL

To make meatballs:
Combine beef, onion, garlic, flour, and seasonings in a bowl. With your hands or a spoon, mix to blend thoroughly. Form into small walnut-sized balls. Heat oil in a skillet. Brown meatballs on all sides. Remove meatballs from skillet.
To make curry sauce:
Melt margarine in skillet. Add onions and garlic powder. While stirring, cook over low heat until onions are soft. Stir in curry powder. Add re-

maining ingredients. Stir to dissolve bouillon cube and blend mixture. Add meatballs. Cover and simmer for 10 minutes.

Yield: 4 servings
Exchange: 1¾ high-fat meat
Calories: 178
Carbohydrates: 2

Eric's Chicken Wings

3	chicken wings	3
1 T.	vegetable oil	15 mL
2 T.	brandy	30 mL
2 T.	water	30 mL
1 T.	soy sauce	15 mL
1 t.	peanut butter	5 mL
1 T.	boiling water	15 mL
½ t.	Worcestershire sauce	2 mL

First clean the chicken wings; then cut them at the joints. Discard wing ends. In a small skillet, brown the wings in the vegetable oil. Add the brandy, 1 T. (15 mL) of the water, and the soy sauce. Cover and cook over medium heat for 15 minutes. Combine the peanut butter and the 1 T. (15 mL) of boiling water in a small bowl. Stir to dissolve peanut butter; then add Worcestershire sauce. Pour over chicken wings. Cover and continue cooking for 7 to 10 minutes. When I was writing the *Diabetic Gourmet Cookbook*, my son, Eric, developed this recipe. It's marvellous as either a snack or an appetizer.

Yield: 1 serving
Exchange: 1 medium-fat meat
Calories: 79
Carbohydrates: 1

Sweet and Sour Pork

4 oz.	pork cubes (fat removed)	120 g
1 t.	soy sauce	5 mL
1 T.	cornstarch	15 mL
2 T.	olive oil	30 mL
½	onion, cut in pieces	½
dash	ground ginger	dash
¼ c.	pineapple chunks, in their own juice	60 mL
1 T.	cold water	15 mL
2 t.	white vinegar	10 mL
2 t.	granulated sugar replacement	10 mL
1 t.	cornstarch	5 mL

Combine pork cubes and soy sauce in a bowl. Stir or toss to coat pork cubes with the soy sauce. Dredge the pork cubes in the 1 T. (15 mL) cornstarch, shaking off any excess. Heat the olive oil in a skillet or wok. Brown the pork cubes. Add the onion and ground ginger. Stir-fry until onions are soft. Add pineapple chunks and juice. While stirring, cook for 1 minute. Combine water, vinegar, sugar replacement, and the 1 t. (5 mL) of cornstarch in shaker bottle; then shake to mix. Pour over pork cubes. While stirring, cook until mixture becomes clear and thickens. I use an Iowa chop (a double-thick chop) for my pork cubes.

Yield: 4 servings
Exchange: 1 lean-meat, 1 fat, ¼ starch/bread
Calories: 113
Carbohydrates: 4

Cheese and Rice Balls

1 c.	cooked rice	250 mL
¼ c.	grated Romano cheese	60 mL
¼ c.	grated Parmesan cheese	60 mL
1	egg, beaten	1
1 t.	horseradish	5 mL

Combine all ingredients; then stir to blend thoroughly. Form into eight balls. In a skillet sprayed with vegetable oil, sauté until lightly browned.

Yield: 8 servings
Exchange, 1 serving: ½ medium-fat meat, ¼ starch/bread
Calories, 1 serving: 59
Carbohydrates, 1 serving: 4

Cottage Cheese Snack

½ c.	low-calorie creamed cottage cheese	125 mL
1	apple, chopped	1
1 t.	cinnamon	5 mL
dash	nutmeg	dash

Combine all ingredients in a bowl. Stir to blend. If desired, cover tightly and refrigerate. This tastes better if you make it the day before so that you can allow the flavors to mingle.

Yield: 2 servings
Exchange, 1 serving: ½ fruit, ½ skim milk
Calories, 1 serving: 71
Carbohydrates, 1 serving: 9

Showcase Meatballs

1 lb.	lean ground beef	500 g
2	eggs	2
⅓ c.	dry breadcrumbs	90 mL
3 T.	skim milk	45 mL
2 t.	onion flakes	10 mL
½ t.	sage	2 mL
dash each	salt and pepper	dash each
2 T.	vegetable oil	30 mL

You can freeze these little beauties and then reheat them for a snack to eat any time of the day. First, mix together beef, eggs, breadcrumbs, milk, onion flakes, sage, salt, and pepper. Then shape into 36 small balls, using damp hands. Heat oil in a skillet. Fry meatballs until browned, rotating the skillet to keep the balls from sticking. Drain. Cool and store in freezer. To reheat: Add desired number of meatballs to a saucepan of boiling bouillon or salted water, and cook for 5 to 7 minutes.

Yield: 36 servings
Exchange, 1 serving: ½ lean meat
Calories, 1 serving: 30
Carbohydrates, 1 serving: 1

Mexican Meatballs

1 lb.	ground beef	500 g
2	eggs	2
⅓ c.	dry bread crumbs	90 mL
2 T.	skim milk	30 mL
1 t.	onion flakes	5 mL
1 env.	Mexican-style dry flavoring mix	1 env.
2 T.	vegetable oil	30 mL

These meatballs can be quickly reheated. Combine beef, eggs, bread crumbs, milk, onion flakes, and Mexican-flavoring mix. Shape into 36 very small balls, using damp hands. Heat oil in a skillet. Fry meatballs until browned, rotating the skillet to keep the balls from sticking. Drain. Cool and store in freezer. To reheat: Add desired number of meatballs to a saucepan of boiling bouillon or salted water and cook for 5 to 7 minutes.

Yield: 36 servings
Exchange, 1 serving: ½ lean meat
Calories, 1 serving: 29
Carbohydrates, 1 serving: 1

Steak Tartare

¼ lb.	sirloin steak (fat and bone removed)	120 g
1 t.	capers	5 mL
1 t.	minced onion	5 mL
½ t.	Dijon-style mustard	2 mL
⅛ t.	white vinegar	½ mL
	salt, pepper, and parsley to taste	

Grind steak twice or chop fine in food processor. Place ground steak in a flat bowl or pie plate. Top with capers, onion, mustard, and vinegar. With two forks, toss meat to incorporate ingredients. Sprinkle with desired amounts of salt, pepper, and parsley. Toss meat lightly. Serve immediately. This makes a marvellous afternoon snack.

Yield: 2 servings
Exchange: 2 medium-fat meat
Calories: 130
Carbohydrates: negligible

Sweet Pork Balls

1 lb.	lean ground pork	500 g
2 t.	granulated sugar replacement	10 mL
1 t.	ground sage	5 mL
¼ t.	nutmeg	1 mL
⅛ t.	crushed fennel seed	½ mL

Combine all ingredients in a bowl, and mix thoroughly. Shape into 40 small balls, using damp hands. Heat a large kettle of salted water to boiling. Drop the pork balls into the water. While stirring, boil until balls are light grey and firm. Remove from water with a slotted spoon. Drain thoroughly. Place the pork balls in small batches in a skillet. Rotating skillet to prevent sticking, fry over low heat until pork balls are browned. Drain. Cool and store in freezer. To reheat: Add desired number of pork balls to a saucepan of boiling bouillon or salted water, and cook for 5 to 7 minutes.

Yield: 40 servings
Exchange, 1 serving: ¼ medium-fat meat
Calories, 1 serving: 19
Carbohydrates, 1 serving: negligible

Veal Patty

2 oz.	veal patty	60 g
1 T.	dry bread crumbs	15 mL
1 T.	vegetable oil	15 mL
2 t.	natural butter-flavored mix	10 mL
	salt and pepper to taste	

Flatten patty to ¼ in. (8 mm). Dampen slightly with water. Press the bread crumbs on both sides of patty. Place on a covered plate in refrigerator for at least 30 minutes. Heat oil in a skillet until a drop of water will sizzle. Now add veal patty and quickly brown both sides. Sprinkle patty with butter-flavored mix. Reduce heat, cover, and cook for 2 minutes.

Yield: 1 serving
Exchange: 2 lean meat, ⅓ starch/bread
Calories: 136
Carbohydrates: 5

Pork Puffs

¾ c.	finely diced cooked pork	190 mL
3 T.	finely cut chives or onion	45 mL
1 t.	finely snipped parsley	5 mL
	salt and pepper to taste	
¾ c.	all-purpose flour	190 mL
½ c.	warm water	125 mL
2 t.	vegetable oil	10 mL
1	egg white, stiffly beaten	1
	deep fat for frying	

Combine pork, chives, parsley, salt, and pepper in a bowl. Stir to mix. Combine flour, water, and vegetable oil in a bowl or blender; then beat into a smooth batter. Fold in pork mixture until blended. Fold in stiffly beaten egg white. Drop by tablespoons into hot oil (365 °F or 180 °C). Fry until golden brown. Drain thoroughly.

Yield: 20 servings
Exchange: ⅓ medium-fat meat, ¼ starch/bread
Calories: 45
Carbohydrates: 4

Parmigiana Ham

2 oz.	ham slice (fully cooked)	60 g
1 T.	skim milk	15 mL
1 T.	dry bread crumbs	15 mL
1 T.	sunflower oil	15 mL
½ oz.	low-fat mozzarella cheese slice	15 g
2 T.	canned pizza sauce	30 mL

Dip ham slice in skim milk. Pat dry bread crumbs on both sides of the ham slice. Heat oil in skillet; then add ham slice. Brown on both sides. Top the ham slice with mozzarella cheese slice and pizza sauce. Cover and heat until cheese is melted.

Yield: 1 serving
Exchange: 2 high-fat meat, 2 fat, ⅓ starch/bread
Calories: 327
Carbohydrates: 5

Shrimp Delight

1 T.	minced onion	15 mL
1 T.	snipped fresh parsley	15 mL
1 T.	minced green pepper	15 mL
⅓ c.	thinly sliced mushrooms	90 mL
½ c.	skim milk	125 mL
2 t.	all-purpose flour	10 mL
dash each	salt, pepper, nutmeg	dash each
½ c.	cooked shrimp	125 mL
2 slices	toasted bread	2 slices

In a skillet sprayed with vegetable oil, sauté onion, parsley, green pepper, and mushrooms until mushrooms are tender. Combine milk and flour in a cup or shaker bottle. Stir or shake to blend. Pour over vegetables. Add dash of salt, pepper, and nutmeg. Then add shrimp. While stirring, cook until mixture is thickened. Spoon over toast.

Yield: 2 servings
Exchange, 1 serving: 1 starch/bread, 1 lean meat, ¼ skim milk
Calories, 1 serving: 175
Carbohydrates, 1 serving: 20

Scalloped Crab

1 c.	crab meat	250 mL
½ c.	soda-cracker crumbs	125 mL
2 t.	low-calorie margarine	10 mL
⅓ c.	skim milk	90 mL
	salt and pepper to taste	

Arrange a layer of crab on the bottom of a baking dish sprayed with vegetable oil. Sprinkle cracker crumbs over the top. Dot with the margarine. Pour in milk and then sprinkle with salt and pepper. Bake at 375 °F (190 °C) for 15 to 20 minutes or until milk is completely absorbed.

Yield: 2 servings
Exchange, 1 serving: 1½ starch/bread, 1 medium-fat meat
Calories, 1 serving: 205
Carbohydrates, 1 serving: 20

Fried Oysters

1 T.	all-purpose flour	15 mL
2 T.	soda-cracker crumbs, very fine	30 mL
6	oysters	6
1 T.	low-calorie margarine	15 mL

Combine flour and cracker crumbs in a small bowl. Roll oysters in crumb-flour mixture. Melt margarine in small skillet. Then sauté oysters until golden brown.

Yield: 1 serving
Exchange: 1 medium-fat meat, 1 starch/bread, 1 fat
Calories: 208
Carbohydrates: 14

Shrimp Egg Rolls

Filling:

5	dried Chinese mushrooms	5
⅛ in.	gingerroot	5 mm
8 oz.	cooked shrimp	250 g
2 cloves	garlic	2 cloves
1	leek, cut in pieces	1
2	carrots, cut in pieces	2
2 T.	olive oil	30 mL
1 c.	sliced water chestnuts	250 mL
2 c.	bean sprouts	500 mL
2 T.	soy sauce	30 mL
½ t.	salt	2 mL
¼ t.	black pepper	1 mL
1 T.	cornstarch	15 mL
1 T.	cold water	15 mL
20	egg-roll wrappers	20
1	egg, slightly beaten	1
	deep fat for frying	

Remove hard stems from mushrooms; then discard. Soak mushrooms in very hot water for about 20 minutes or until soft. Drain. Slice thin. Using steel blade of food processor, with machine running, drop ginger-root through feeder tube. Process until minced. Sprinkle over shrimp and set aside. With food processor running, drop in garlic, leek, and carrot pieces. Process until coarsely chopped. Heat the olive oil in a wok or skillet. Then add the chopped garlic, leek, and carrot, along with the sliced mushrooms, sliced water chestnuts, bean sprouts, soy sauce, salt, and pepper. Stir-fry for 30 seconds; then cover and cook for 30 more seconds. Add shrimp. Stir-fry until shrimp is pink. Combine cornstarch and cold water in a small bowl. Stir to blend. Pour into shrimp mixture. While stirring, cook lightly until mixture thickens. Remove mixture from wok and cool slightly. Place 2 T. (30 mL) of filling in center of each egg roll. Fold the corner of egg roll over filling; then fold in the two side corners. Brush the remaining corner with slightly beaten egg. Roll up. Place on lightly floured surface until ready to fry. Fry in deep fat at 375 °F (190 °C) until golden brown. Serve with Sweet Sauce.

Sweet Sauce:

2 (4 oz.) jars	apricot baby food	2 (128 g) jars
3 T.	white vinegar	45 mL
3 T.	cold water	45 mL
1 T.	granulated sugar replacement	15 mL
2 t.	cornstarch	10 mL

Combine all ingredients in a saucepan. Stir to blend. While stirring, cook sauce over low heat until it thickens. Even though it may seem complex, this is an easy food-processor recipe.

Yield: 20 servings
Exchange, 1 serving: ¼ lean meat; $1/_5$ fruit
Calories, 1 serving: 16
Carbohydrates, 1 serving: 3

Tuna Casserole

7-oz. can	tuna in water	198-g can
10-oz. can	cream of mushroom soup	258-g can
2 c.	crushed potato chips	500 mL
2 T.	minced chives	30 mL

Combine all ingredients in a bowl. Toss to mix. Turn into a casserole or baking dish, sprayed with vegetable oil. Bake at 375 °F (190 °C) for 30 to 35 minutes.

Yield: 6 servings
Exchange, 1 serving: 1 starch/bread, ½ lean meat
Calories, 1 serving: 110
Carbohydrates, 1 serving: 10

Salmon Patties

1-lb. can	salmon	456-g can
¼ c.	dry bread crumbs	60 mL
¼ c.	ketchup	60 mL
¼ c.	snipped chives	60 mL
1	egg	1

Drain salmon thoroughly and then remove any bones or skin. Combine with remaining ingredients in a bowl. Stir to mix. Form into eight patties. Fry until browned on both sides in a skillet sprayed with vegetable oil.

Yield: 8 servings
Exchange, 1 serving: 1 medium-fat meat, ¼ starch/bread
Calories, 1 serving: 105
Carbohydrates, 1 serving: 4

Chinese Egg Cakes

3	dried Chinese mushrooms	3
1 cube	beef bouillon	1 cube
1 c.	hot water	250 mL
½ lb.	bulk pork sausage, cooked and drained	250 g
½ c.	finely chopped onions	125 mL
1 c.	bean sprouts	250 mL
2 T.	soy sauce	30 mL
¼ t.	salt	1 mL
4	eggs, slightly beaten	4
3 T.	sunflower oil	45 mL
1 t.	cornstarch	5 mL
1 T.	cold water	15 mL

Remove hard stems from mushrooms and discard. Soak mushrooms in very hot water for about 20 minutes or until soft. Drain. Slice thin. Dissolve bouillon cube in the 1 c. (250 mL) of hot water. Combine mushrooms, pork sausage, onions, bean sprouts, 1 T. (15 mL) of the soy sauce, the salt, ⅓ c. (90 mL) of the beef bouillon, and the eggs in a bowl. Stir to mix. Heat the sunflower oil in a wok. Spoon egg mixture into hot oil, about 1 T. (15 mL) at a time. Do not crowd pan. Fry egg cakes until golden brown. Transfer to warmed platter. Now combine cornstarch and the 1 T. (15 mL) of cold water in a small bowl. Stir to blend. Combine the remaining beef bouillon, the remaining soy sauce, and the corn-starch mixture in a small saucepan and then cook over low heat until clear and thickened. Pour over hot egg cakes to serve.

Yield: 20 servings
Exchange, 1 serving: ½ medium-fat meat, ⅓ fat
Calories, 1 serving: 50
Carbohydrates, 1 serving: 2

Scallop Bake

2 lbs.	scallops	1 kg
1 c.	water	250 mL
⅓ c.	lemon juice	90 mL
2 c.	thinly sliced mushrooms	500 mL
1	green pepper, diced	1
⅓ c.	finely chopped yellow onion	90 mL
3 T.	all-purpose flour	45 mL
½ t.	salt	2 mL
⅛ t.	black pepper	½ mL
½ c.	diced Swiss cheese	125 mL
¼ c.	grated Romano cheese	60 mL
¾ c.	prepared nondairy whipped topping paprika	190 mL

Wash and drain scallops. Bring water and lemon juice to a boil in a medium-sized saucepan. Add scallops, mushrooms, green pepper, and onion. Reduce heat and simmer on LOW for 8 minutes. Remove from heat. Pour a small amount of the scallop liquid from the saucepan into a blender or small bowl. Add the flour, salt, and pepper to the liquid. Blend until smooth. Pour back into saucepan. While stirring, cook until mixture has thickened. Stir in cheeses. While continuing to stir, cook over low heat until cheeses have melted. Remove from heat. Fold in prepared nondairy whipped topping. Divide mixture evenly among 10 individual baking dishes. Sprinkle with paprika. Then broil until browned. This is an excellent appetizer or snack.

Yield: 10 servings
Exchange, 1 serving: 2 lean meat, ½ starch/bread
Calories, 1 serving: 147
Carbohydrates, 1 serving: 7

Sautéed Salmon

½	onion, thinly sliced	½
4 oz.	boned salmon steak	120 g
1 T.	all-purpose flour	15 mL
	salt and pepper to taste	

Sauté onion in a skillet that has been sprayed with vegetable oil. When onion is evenly browned, remove and set aside. Recoat skillet with vegetable-oil spray. Flour the salmon steak on both sides; next, season with salt and pepper. Cook until fish flakes easily when tested with a fork or toothpick. Transfer to warm plate and cover with onions.

Yield: 1 serving
Exchange, 1 serving: 2 medium-fat meat
Calories, 1 serving: 172
Carbohydrates, 1 serving: 3

Swordfish Amandine

2 T.	chopped almonds	30 mL
4 oz.	swordfish steak	120 g
1 t.	chopped parsley	5 mL
1 t.	lemon juice	5 mL
1 T.	dry sherry	15 mL

Brown almonds in a skillet sprayed with vegetable oil. Set aside. Place swordfish in a metal pie pan. Spray fish with vegetable oil. Combine parsley, lemon juice, and sherry in a small bowl. Spoon half of this sauce over the fish. Broil for 10 minutes, basting lightly after 5 minutes. Turn fish and then coat with vegetable-oil spray again. Spoon half of the remaining sauce over fish. Replace in broiler and cook for 10 minutes more, basting after 5 minutes. Place on warmed plate, and garnish with almonds.

Yield: 1 serving
Exchange: 2 high-fat meat
Calories: 217
Carbohydrates: 3

Beer-Batter Fried Cheese

1 lb.	Swiss cheese	500 g
2	eggs, slightly beaten	2
⅔ c.	nonalcoholic beer	180 mL
¼ t.	Tabasco sauce	1 mL
1 c.	all-purpose flour	250 mL
½ t.	salt	2 mL
1 T.	vegetable oil	15 mL
	deep fat for frying	

Cut cheese into 2 in. × 1 in. strips that are ½ in. thick (5 cm × 2.5 cm × 1.25 cm). Combine eggs, beer and Tabasco sauce in a bowl; next, slowly beat in the flour, salt, and vegetable oil. Dip cheese strips into beer batter. Fry in hot oil at 365 °F (184 °C) until golden brown.

Yield: 10 servings
Exchange, 1 serving: 2 high-fat meat, ½ starch/bread
Calories, 1 serving: 224
Carbohydrates, 1 serving: 8

Salmon-Stuffed Eggs

5	eggs, hard-cooked	5
¼ c.	drained and boned salmon	60 mL
¼ c.	cream cheese, softened	60 mL
	salt and pepper to taste	

Shell eggs and cut in half lengthwise. Carefully remove yolks to a bowl. Set whites aside. Add salmon, cream cheese, salt, and pepper to yolks. Beat until smooth. Stuff egg whites with mixture.

Yield: 10 servings
Exchange, 1 serving: ⅔ medium-fat meat
Calories, 1 serving: 61
Carbohydrates, 1 serving: negligible

Breads

Mushroom and Onion Bread

1 c.	skim milk	250 mL
1 T.	finely chopped onion	15 mL
1 large	mushroom, finely chopped	1 large
1 env.	dry yeast	1 env.
1 t.	granulated sugar	5 mL
¼ c.	warm water	60 mL
1 t.	salt	5 mL
1 T.	sunflower oil	15 mL
3 c.	all-purpose flour	750 mL

Combine skim milk, onion, and mushroom in a small saucepan. Heat just to boiling. Cover and allow to cook to lukewarm. Combine yeast and sugar in the warm water. Stir to dissolve yeast. Add to milk mixture. Beat in salt and sunflower oil. Add 1½ c. (375 mL) of the flour. Beat until dough is a smooth batter. Work in remaining flour. Turn out onto lightly floured surface; then knead for 10 minutes. Cover and allow to rise until double in size. Punch down and form into a loaf. Place in a large loaf pan sprayed with vegetable oil. Cover and allow to rise. Then bake at 375 °F (190 °C) for 25 to 30 minutes or until golden brown.

Yield: 16 servings
Exchange, 1 serving: 1 starch/bread
Calories, 1 serving: 84
Carbohydrates, 1 serving: 17

Orange Bread

1 c.	orange juice	250 mL
1 env.	dry yeast	1 env.
1 T.	low-calorie margarine, melted	15 mL
1 t.	honey	5 mL
1 t.	salt	5 mL
1 t.	orange rind	5 mL
3 c.	all-purpose flour	750 mL

Heat orange juice until lukewarm. Stir in yeast, margarine, and honey. Allow yeast to soften; then stir to dissolve completely. Add salt and orange rind. Next, add flour. Mix well. Allow to rise until doubled in size. Turn out onto lightly floured board; then knead for 10 minutes. Form into a loaf. Place in lightly oiled loaf pan. Cover and allow to rise. Bake at 375 °F (190 °C) for 30 to 40 minutes. This bread is especially good with ham.

Yield: 16 servings
Exchange, 1 serving: 1 starch/bread
Calories, 1 serving: 80
Carbohydrates, 1 serving: 16

Corn Bread

¾ c.	cornmeal	190 mL
1 c.	all-purpose flour	250 mL
¼ c.	granulated sugar replacement	60 mL
1½ T.	baking powder	22 mL
½ t.	salt	2 mL
1	egg, well-beaten	1
1 c.	skim milk	250 mL
1 T.	vegetable oil	15 mL

Mix and sift the dry ingredients. Combine all ingredients in a mixing bowl. Beat just to blend. Pour into an 8 in. (20 cm) baking pan. Then bake at 350 °F (175 °C) for 20 to 25 minutes or until done.

Yield: 16 servings
Exchange, 1 serving: ¾ starch/bread
Calories, 1 serving: 62
Carbohydrates, 1 serving: 12

Graham Bread

1 env.	yeast	1 env.	
¼ c.	lukewarm water	60 mL	
2 t.	honey	10 mL	
2 c.	warm water	500 mL	
¼ c.	granulated brown-sugar replacement	60 mL	
2 T.	vegetable oil	30 mL	
2 t.	salt	10 mL	
½ c.	all-purpose flour	125 mL	
1 c.	soy flour	250 mL	
4½ c.	graham flour	1125 mL	

Soften yeast in lukewarm water; then allow to stand for 5 minutes. Stir in honey. Combine the 2 c. (500 mL) of water, the brown-sugar replacement, oil, salt, all-purpose flour, and soy flour in a large mixing bowl. Beat to blend. Gradually beat in graham flour. Turn out onto lightly floured surface. Knead in any remaining flour. Cover and allow to rise until doubled in size. Knead slightly. Allow to rest for 5 minutes. Then form into two loaves. Place in lightly oiled loaf pans. Cover and allow to rise until doubled in size. Bake at 400 °F (200 °C) for 50 minutes or until done.

Yield: 30 servings
Exchange, 1 serving: 1 starch/bread
Calories, 1 serving: 83
Carbohydrates, 1 serving: 17

Blue-Cheese Bread

1 env.	yeast	1 env.	
1 t.	granulated sugar	5 mL	
¼ c.	warm water	60 mL	
¾ c.	skim milk	190 mL	
¼ c.	blue cheese	60 mL	
¼ c.	finely snipped chives	60 mL	
1 T.	sunflower oil	15 mL	
2½ c.	bread flour	625 mL	
½ c.	rye flour	125 mL	

Sprinkle yeast and sugar over warm water in bowl. Allow to soften; then stir to dissolve. In a blender, combine milk and blue cheese. Blend on

HIGH until mixture is creamy. Pour into a large mixing bowl. Stir in yeast-sugar mixture, chives, and oil. Add half of the bread flour; then beat into a batter. Continue beating, gradually adding remaining bread flour and the rye flour. Cover and allow to rise until doubled in size. Now grease two 8 in. (20 cm) baking pans. Divide dough in half. Form each half of the dough into the botom of the baking pans. Cover and allow to rise until doubled in size. Bake at 400 °F (200 °C) for 30 minutes or until done. Then immediately remove from pans and allow to cool on racks.

Yield: 24 servings
Exchange, 1 serving: ¾ starch/bread
Calories, 1 serving: 60
Carbohydrates, 1 serving: 12

Amaretto Tea Bread

2 bags	amaretto tea	2 bags
1 c.	boiling water	250 mL
1 env.	dry yeast	1 env.
3¼ c.	all-purpose flour	810 mL
1 T.	vegetable oil	15 mL
1 t.	salt	5 mL
1 t.	granulated sugar	5 mL

Allow tea bags to steep in the boiling water until the tea becomes very dark and cool. Sprinkle yeast over tea. Stir and then allow to soften for 5 minutes. Combine flour, oil, salt, and sugar in food processor with steel blade. With food processor running, pour yeast-tea mixture through the feeder tube. Dough will ball and clean sides of processor bowl. Allow to process for 30 to 40 seconds. Then transfer dough to bowl or flat surface. Cover loosely with plastic wrap. Allow dough to rise until double in size. Lightly oil (or spray with vegetable oil) a loaf pan. Knead dough (dough will be slightly sticky) for about 10 minutes. Form into a loaf; then place in loaf pan. Do not cover. Place in warm draft-free area until doubled in size. Bake at 400 °F (200 °C) for 35 to 40 minutes or until done. Since breads made in the food processor are heavier but very flavorful, they should be cut into very thin slices.

Yield: 16 servings
Exchange, 1 serving: 1 starch/bread
Calories, 1 serving: 85
Carbohydrates, 1 serving: 15

Quick French Bread

1 env.	yeast	1 env.
1¼ c.	warm water	310 mL
1 t.	granulated sugar	5 mL
1 t.	salt	5 mL
1 T.	vegetable oil	15 mL
3¼ c.	all-purpose flour	810 mL

Sprinkle yeast over warm water in a large mixing bowl. Stir to blend.
Allow to rest for 5 minutes. Add sugar, salt, oil, and half of the flour.
Beat until smooth with an electric mixer. Stir in remaining flour. Cover
the bowl with plastic wrap. Allow to rise until doubled in size. Now
lightly grease a cookie sheet. Form dough into an 18 in. (45 cm) roll.
Place on cookie sheet. Do not cover. Allow to rise until doubled in size.
Just before baking, brush lightly with cold water. Then bake at 350 °F
(175 °C) for 25 to 30 minutes or until done.

Yield: 24 servings
Exchange, 1 serving: ¾ starch/bread
Calories, 1 serving: 57
Carbohydrates, 1 serving: 11

Buttermilk Bread

1 c.	buttermilk	250 mL
½ c.	wheat-barley cereal granules	125 mL
2 c.	biscuit mix	500 mL
1 t.	cinnamon	5 mL
⅛ t.	mace	½ mL
⅛ t.	ginger	½ mL
½ c.	water	125 mL

Combine buttermilk and cereal in a bowl. Stir to mix. Allow to rest for
at least an hour or until cereal is soft. Combine biscuit mix, cinnamon,
mace, and ginger in a mixing bowl. Stir to blend. Then add buttermilk-
cereal mixture and water. Stir to mix. Turn dough into a lightly vegeta-
ble-oiled loaf pan. Bake at 350 °F (175 °C) for an hour or until done.

Yield: 12 servings
Exchange, 1 serving: 1 starch/bread
Calories, 1 serving: 85
Carbohydrates, 1 serving: 17

Everyday Nut Bread

2 c.	biscuit mix	500 mL
⅓ c.	granulated brown-sugar replacement	90 mL
1 c.	skim milk	250 mL
1	egg, well-beaten	1
1 T.	low-calorie margarine, melted	15 mL
½ c.	chopped pecan halves	125 mL

Combine all ingredients in a mixing bowl. Stir well to blend. Pour into a well-greased loaf pan. Bake at 350 °F (175 °C) for an hour or until cake tester inserted in center comes out clean.

Yield: 16 servings
Exchange, 1 serving: 1 starch/bread
Calories, 1 serving: 88
Carbohydrates, 1 serving: 13

Graham Nut Bread

2 c.	graham flour	500 mL
3 c.	all-purpose flour	750 mL
1 T.	baking soda	15 mL
1 c.	granulated sugar replacement	250 mL
¾ c.	chopped walnuts	190 mL
½ c.	granulated brown-sugar replacement	125 mL
½ t.	salt	2 mL
3 c.	buttermilk	750 mL
2	eggs, well-beaten	2
1 T.	vegetable oil	15 mL
1 t.	vanilla extract	5 mL

Combine dry ingredients in a large mixing bowl. Stir to mix. Add remaining ingredients and beat just to blend. Spread evenly on the bottom of two well-greased loaf pans. Allow to rest for 15 minutes. Then bake at 325 °F (165 °C) for an hour or until done. The graham flour and brown-sugar replacement give this bread its special flavor.

Yield: 26 servings
Exchange, 1 serving: 1½ starch/bread
Calories, 1 serving: 119
Carbohydrates, 1 serving: 21

Cheese Graham Bread

1 env.	dry yeast	1 env.
¼ c.	warm water	60 mL
11-oz. can	cheese soup	312-g can
2 c.	all-purpose flour	500 mL
1 c.	graham flour	250 mL

Sprinkle yeast over warm water in bowl. Stir and then allow to soften for 5 minutes. Combine remaining ingredients in food processor with steel blade. With food processor running, pour yeast-water mixture through the feeder tube. Dough will ball and clean sides of processor bowl. Allow to process for 30 to 40 seconds. Then transfer dough to bowl or flat surface. Cover loosely with plastic wrap. Allow dough to rise until double in size. Lightly oil (or spray with vegetable oil) a loaf pan or casserole dish. Knead dough (dough will be slightly sticky) for about 10 minutes. Form into a loaf; then place in loaf pan or casserole dish. Do not cover. Place in warm draft-free area until doubled in size. Bake at 400 °F (200 °C) for 35 to 40 minutes or until done. I like to bake this bread in an oval casserole dish.

Yield: 16 servings
Exchange, 1 serving: 1¼ starch/bread
Calories, 1 serving: 102
Carbohydrates, 1 serving: 18

Chocolate Bread

1 env.	dry yeast	1 env.
1 c.	warm water	250 mL
2½ c.	all-purpose flour	625 mL
½ c.	unsweetened cocoa	125 mL
½ c.	granulated sugar replacement	125 mL
½ t.	salt	2 mL

Sprinkle yeast over warm water in bowl. Stir and then allow to soften for 5 minutes. Combine remaining ingredients in food processor with steel blade. Process on HIGH to blend. With food processor running, pour yeast-water mixture through the feeder tube. Dough will ball and clean sides of processor bowl. Allow to process for 30 to 40 seconds. Then transfer dough to bowl or flat surface. Cover the dough loosely with plastic wrap. Allow dough to rise until double in size. Lightly oil (or spray with vegetable oil) a loaf pan. Knead dough (dough will be slightly sticky) for about 10 minutes. Form into a loaf; then place in loaf pan. Do not cover. Place in warm draft-free area until doubled in size. Bake at 400 °F (200 °C) for 35 to 40 minutes or until done. This chocolate-flavored yeast bread will melt in your mouth.

Yield: 14 servings
Exchange, 1 serving: 1 starch/bread
Calories, 1 serving: 77
Carbohydrates, 1 serving: 16

Refrigerator Dough

1 env.	dry yeast	1 env.
2 T.	warm water	30 mL
1 c.	skim milk, warmed	250 mL
3 T.	granulated sugar replacement	45 mL
2 t.	granulated sugar	10 mL
1½ t.	salt	7 mL
½ t.	mace	2 mL
2	eggs, well-beaten	2
4 c.	sifted all-purpose flour	1000 mL
¼ c.	low-calorie margarine, melted	60 mL

Sprinkle yeast over bowl of warm water; then allow to soften for 5 minutes. Stir to blend. Combine warmed milk, sugar replacement, sugar, salt, and mace in a large mixing bowl. Next, add softened yeast, eggs, and half of the flour. Beat into a soft sponge dough. While beating, gradually add melted margarine. Allow sponge dough to rest 5 minutes. Then beat in remaining flour. Place in a large lightly oiled bowl, cover, and allow to chill 4 to 6 hours or overnight. This sweet dough can be used in many recipes or baked as a sweet bread. If using the dough for another recipe, follow that recipe's directions at this point. If using it for sweet bread, form into two loaves and place in lightly oiled loaf pans. Then cover with plastic wrap and allow to rise until double in size. Bake at 375 °F (190 °C) for 30 to 35 minutes or until done.

Yield: 24 servings
Exchange, 1 serving: 1¼ starch/bread
Calories, 1 serving: 97
Carbohydrates, 1 serving: 18

Orange-Cranberry-Nut Bread

3 c.	all-purpose flour	750 mL
¾ c.	granulated sugar replacement	190 mL
4 t.	baking powder	20 mL
1 t.	salt	5 mL
½ t.	baking soda	2 mL
1 T.	grated orange peel	15 mL
½ c.	chopped walnuts	125 mL
1½ c.	chopped cranberries	375 mL
½ c.	evaporated skim milk	125 mL
½ c.	orange juice	125 mL
1	egg, slightly beaten	1
2 T.	low-calorie margarine, melted	30 mL

Sift flour, sugar replacement, baking powder, salt, and baking soda together. Next, stir in orange peel, walnuts, and cranberries. In a separate bowl, combine evaporated milk, orange juice, egg, and melted margarine; then beat to blend. Blend egg mixture into flour mixture. Pour into a well-greased 9-in. (23-cm) tube pan. Bake at 350 °F (175 °C) for 50 to 60 minutes or until done.

Yield: 24 servings
Exchange, 1 serving: 1 starch/bread
Calories, 1 serving: 77
Carbohydrates, 1 serving: 14

Tomato Pecan Bread

1 env.	dry yeast	1 env.
¼ c.	warm water	60 mL
½ c.	pecan halves	125 mL
3½ c.	all-purpose flour	810 mL
3 T.	granulated sugar replacement	45 mL
10-oz. can	tomato soup	305-g can

Sprinkle yeast over bowl of warm water. Stir and then allow to soften for 5 minutes. Process pecan halves in a food processor with a steel blade until coarsely chopped. Add remaining ingredients. Process on HIGH to blend. With food processor running, pour yeast-water mixture through the feeder tube. Dough will ball and clean sides of processor bowl. Allow to process for 30 to 40 seconds. Transfer dough to bowl. (This dough is very sticky.) Cover the dough loosely with plastic wrap. Allow dough to rise until double in size. Lightly oil a loaf pan (or use vegetable oil spray). Then turn dough into the loaf pan. Do not cover. Place in warm draft-free area until doubled in size. Bake at 400 °F (200 °C) for 20 minutes. Reduce heat to 375 °F (190 °C) and bake 20 to 25 minutes more or until done. Cut in 13 thin slices; then cut each slice in half. This nutty sweet bread is one of my favorites.

Yield: 26 servings
Exchange, 1 serving: 1 starch/bread
Calories, 1 serving: 81
Carbohydrates, 1 serving: 11

Dried Apricot Bread

2½ c.	biscuit mix	625 mL
½ c.	granulated sugar replacement	125 mL
2 T.	low-calorie margarine	30 mL
¾ c.	dried apricots	190 mL
1 c.	skim milk	250 mL
2	eggs, well-beaten	2

Combine biscuit mix, sugar replacement, and margarine in a mixing bowl. Cut with two forks or a pastry blender until mixture resembles coarse meal. Cut apricots into small pieces. Add apricots to flour mixture. Toss to coat apricot pieces. Now combine milk and eggs. Beat to blend. Add egg mixture to dry ingredients, stirring just until mixed. Spoon or turn batter into well-greased loaf pan. Bake at 350 °F (175 °C) for an hour or until done. This bread is easy to make and freezes in slices extremely well.

Yield: 12 servings
Exchange, 1 serving: 1¼ starch/bread, ⅓ fruit
Calories, 1 serving: 129
Carbohydrates, 1 serving: 24

Tidbits

Danish-Style Meatballs

2 lbs.	lean ground round	1 kg
½ lb.	lean ground pork	250 mL
¾ c.	all-purpose flour	190 mL
¾ c.	evaporated skim milk	190 mL
3	eggs	3
2	onions, cut in pieces	2
2 t.	salt	10 mL
1 t.	granulated sugar replacement	5 mL
½ t.	ground ginger	2 mL

Combine ground round and ground pork in a large bowl. With a spoon or your hands, work until well mixed. Combine remaining ingredients in a food processor with a steel blade or in a blender. Blend until smooth. Pour into meats, and work until completely incorporated. Form into 40 small balls. Heat a large kettle half full of water to boiling. Drop meatballs individually into the boiling water. Do not crowd kettle. When meat is firm and brown, remove with a slotted spoon. To serve: Fry gently in a skillet over low heat until toasted. You can make these meatballs any time and then freeze them in small amounts to be used later.

Yield: 40 servings
Exchange, 1 serving: 1 medium-fat meat
Calories, 1 serving: 64
Carbohydrates, 1 serving: 3

Potato-Crab Nibblers

1 c.	prepared mashed potatoes	250 mL
1 t.	dry minced onion	5 mL
1 t.	Worcestershire sauce	5 mL
⅛ t.	garlic powder	½ mL
7½-oz. can	crab meat, drained and flaked	220-g can
1	egg, slightly beaten	1
½ c.	dry bread crumbs	125 mL
	deep fat for frying	

Combine prepared mashed potatoes, minced onion, Worcestershire sauce, garlic powder, and crab meat in a bowl. Fold to completely blend. Shape into 36 bite-size balls. Dip into beaten egg; then roll in crumbs. Fry in deep fat at 375 °F (190 °C) for about a minute or until golden brown. Drain thoroughly.

Yield: 36 servings
Exchange, 1 serving: ¼ starch/bread
Calories, 1 serving: 16
Carbohydrates, 1 serving: 4

Herbed Cheese on Toast

8 slices	white bread	8 slices
8 oz.	cream cheese, softened	250 g
1 T.	skim milk	15 mL
1 t.	minced onion	5 mL
¼ t.	minced garlic	1 mL
1 t.	thyme	5 mL
1 t.	sweet basil	5 mL
1 t.	dill seed	5 mL
	salt and pepper to taste	

Toast the bread slices. Cut off crusts and cut each bread slice into three finger-shaped pieces. Set aside. Combine remaining ingredients in a food processor or mixing bowl. Beat to blend thoroughly. Then spread mixture on toast fingers.

Yield: 24 servings
Exchange, 1 serving: ¼ starch/bread, ½ fat
Calories, 1 serving: 48
Carbohydrates, 1 serving: 4

Cucumber and Onion Relish

2	cucumbers	2
2	white onions	2
1 t.	salt	5 mL
2 T.	white vinegar	30 mL
¼ c.	water	60 mL
1 env.	aspartame low-calorie sweetener	1 env.

Score the cucumbers with the tines of a fork (do not peel) and then cut off the ends. Remove peel from onions and cut one slice from each end; then discard peel and ends. Using a sharp knife or slicer in a food processor, slice cucumber and onions very thin. Place in a bowl; then sprinkle with salt. Toss to mix. Cover and allow to rest for an hour. Drain off any liquid. Combine vinegar, water, and sweetener in a bowl. Stir to blend. Pour vinegar mixture over cucumbers and onions. Refrigerate until ready to use. To make wilted cucumbers, prepare this at least a day in advance.

Yield: 20 servings
Exchange, 1 serving: negligible
Calories, 1 serving: negligible
Carbohydrates, 1 serving: negligible

Red Cabbage

1 head	red cabbage, thinly shredded	1 head
1 c.	water	250 mL
1 t.	salt	5 mL
½ c.	white vinegar	125 mL
3 env.	aspartame low-calorie sweetener	3 env.

Parboil the cabbage in the salt water until it is tender. Drain thoroughly, squeezing any excess water out with your hands. Place in a bowl with a cover. Add vinegar and sweetener. Then cover and shake to mix. To serve: Reheat and drain. (Refrigerate to keep.) I don't know whether to call this a relish or an appetizer. People seem to like it; so I tend to make it often.

Yield: 40 servings
Exchange, 1 serving: negligible
Calories, 1 serving: negligible
Carbohydrates, 1 serving: negligible

Rolled Pickles

3 large	dill pickles	3 large
3-oz. pkg.	cream cheese, softened	90-g pkg.
2.5-oz. pkg.	pressed corned beef	71-g pkg.

Dry off any moisture from pickles with paper towels. Cut off ends. Spread cheese around outside of pickles. Divide pressed corned beef into three parts. Separate slices of beef and wrap them around each pickle. Cut each pickle into 10 slices. Refrigerate until ready to serve. If you can't take salt, then this isn't the recipe for you. My mother used to make these with crock dills.

Yield: 30 servings
Exchange, 1 serving: ¼ lean meat
Calories, 1 serving: 14
Carbohydrates, 1 serving: negligible

Grilled Scallops

24	bay scallops	24
3 T.	olive oil	45 mL
¼ c.	cider vinegar	60 mL
2 cloves	garlic, minced	2 cloves
2 t.	black pepper	10 mL
2 large	red bell peppers	2 large
12 slices	bacon	12 slices

Combine scallops, oil, vinegar, garlic, and black pepper in a bowl. Cover and marinate for 24 hours. Peel and seed bell peppers, and then cut them into 2-in. (5-cm) squares. Place bell-pepper squares in a saucepan of boiling water. Reduce heat and allow to simmer for about a minute or until pepper is crispy-tender. Now cut bacon in half crosswise. Fry it over low heat until partially cooked but still limp. Place on a paper-lined plate to drain. Wrap one scallop and one red-pepper square in a bacon strip. Skewer with bamboo sticks or poultry pins. Grill until bacon is crisp.

Yield: 24 servings
Exchange, 1 serving: ½ medium-fat meat
Calories, 1 serving: 36
Carbohydrates, 1 serving: negligible

Water-Chestnut Nibbles

16	whole water chestnuts	16
¼ c.	soy sauce	60 mL
4 slices	bacon	4 slices

Drain water chestnuts thoroughly. Marinate in soy sauce for 30 to 40 minutes. Cut bacon in half both lengthwise and crosswise. Wrap a chestnut in each small slice of bacon. Secure with a toothpick. Arrange on a cookie sheet. Then bake at 400 °F (200 °C) for 20 minutes. Or refrigerate to store, and reheat for 5 minutes before serving. This is a pop-in-the-mouth type of snack or appetizer.

Yield: 16 servings
Exchange, 1 serving: ¼ fat
Calories, 1 serving: 10
Carbohydrates, 1 serving: 1

Pickled Eggs

12	eggs	12
1½ c.	white vinegar	375 mL
½ c.	water	125 mL
¾ c.	granulated sugar replacement	190 mL
1 t.	salt	5 mL
6 whole	cloves	6 whole
1 large	bay leaf	1 large
1	onion, sliced	1

Cover eggs with cold water in a saucepan, bring to a boil, reduce heat, and allow to simmer for 20 minutes. Drain immediately; then run cold water over eggs for several minutes. Peel eggs and then place in a deep glass bowl or glass jar (do not use plastic or metal). Combine vinegar, water, sugar replacement, salt, cloves, and bay leaf in a saucepan. Bring to a boil, reduce heat, and simmer for 5 minutes. Pour hot vinegar mixture over eggs, making sure eggs are completely covered. Lay onion slices on top of mixture. Cover tightly and refrigerate for at least three days. Serve whole or cut in halves.

Yield: 12 servings
Exchange, 1 serving: 1 medium-fat meat
Calories, 1 serving: 80
Carbohydrates, 1 serving: negligible

Pickled Fish

2 lbs.	raw catfish, cut in steaks	1 kg
½ c.	salt	125 mL
1 qt.	cold water	1 L
3 c.	cider vinegar	750 mL
1 c.	lemon juice	250 mL
1 c.	granulated sugar replacement	250 mL
4	bay leaves	4
12 small	dried red peppers	12 small
1 t.	peppercorns	5 mL
3	yellow onions, sliced	3

Wash fish under cold running water. Place in a glass bowl or jar (do not use plastic or metal). Dissolve salt in water. Pour over fish. Allow fish to soak in brine at least 12 hours. Drain. Meanwhile, combine vinegar, lemon juice, sugar replacement, bay leaves, red peppers, and peppercorns in a saucepan. Bring to a boil, reduce heat, and simmer for 5 minutes. Cool completely. Pour cooled vinegar mixture over the fish. Add onions and cover tightly. Tip bowl or jar occasionally to keep fish from packing into a solid. Refrigerate 2 weeks before serving.

Yield: 15 servings
Exchange, 1 serving: 1½ lean meat
Calories, 1 serving: 66
Carbohydrates, 1 serving: negligible

Onion-Cheese Ball

8 oz.	cream cheese, softened	250 g
1 env.	dry onion-soup mix	1 env.

Combine ingredients in a bowl. With an electric mixer, beat to thoroughly blend. Chill until you can work it with your hands. Form into a ball. I frequently keep this in a bowl for the family to nibble.

Yield: 40 servings
Exchange, 1 serving: ½ fat
Calories, 1 serving: 24
Carbohydrates, 1 serving: 2

Pastrami Roll-Ups

3-oz. pkg.	cream cheese, softened	90-g pkg.
2 T.	red wine	30 mL
1 T.	minced onion	15 mL
2 t.	horseradish	10 mL
dash	Worcestershire sauce	dash
12 slices	pressed pastrami	12 slices

Combine cream cheese, wine, onion, horseradish, and Worcestershire sauce in a bowl. Beat until blended and fluffy. Carefully unfold slices of pastrami, and flatten. Spread cheese mixture on pastrami slices. Then roll up as tight as possible. These freeze very well. Take them out of the freezer at least 15 minutes before serving time.

Yield: 12 servings
Exchange, 1 serving: ½ medium-fat meat
Calories, 1 serving: 33
Carbohydrates, 1 serving: 3

Braunschweiger Ball

1 lb.	braunschweiger	500 g
8 oz.	cream cheese, softened	250 g
¼ c.	low-calorie salad dressing	60 mL
2 T.	dill-pickle juice	30 mL
1 t.	Worcestershire sauce	5 mL
¼ t.	garlic powder	1 mL
⅛ t.	hot sauce	½ mL
⅓ c.	finely chopped dill pickle	90 mL
¼ c.	finely chopped onion	60 mL

In a mixing bowl, combine braunschweiger, cream cheese, salad dressing, dill-pickle juice, Worcestershire sauce, garlic powder, and hot sauce. Beat until well blended. Stir in dill pickle and onion. Refrigerate until mixture is cool enough to handle. Then form into a ball. Refrigerate until ready to serve. This dish is a German favorite.

Yield: 20 servings
Exchange, 1 serving: ½ high-fat meat
Calories, 1 serving: 56
Carbohydrates, 1 serving: 2

Parsley-Shrimp Ball

2 (6 oz.) pkgs.	frozen cooked shrimp	2 (170 g) pkgs.
8 oz.	cream cheese, softened	250 g
3 T.	finely chopped celery	45 mL
1 clove	garlic, minced	1 clove
1 t.	soy sauce	5 mL
¼ t.	hot sauce	1 mL
½ c.	finely snipped fresh parsley	125 mL

Thaw, drain, and finely chop the shrimp. Combine shrimp, cream cheese, celery, garlic, soy sauce, and hot sauce in a bowl. Beat to blend. Chill until you can work it with your hands. Form into a ball. Then roll in finely snipped parsley.

Yield: 40 servings
Exchange, 1 serving: ⅓ medium-fat meat
Calories, 1 serving: 24
Carbohydrates, 1 serving: negligible

Cheese-Bacon Crispies

¼ c.	low-calorie margarine, softened	60 mL
¼ lb.	Cheddar cheese, grated	250 g
1 t.	Worcestershire sauce	5 mL
¼ t.	Dijon-style mustard	1 mL
2 T.	bacon bits	30 mL
⅔ c.	all-purpose flour	180 mL

Combine margarine, cheese, Worcestershire sauce, and mustard in a mixing bowl. Beat to blend. Add bacon bits and flour. Mix well. Form into a 1 in. (1.25 cm)-thick roll. Wrap in waxed paper and refrigerate overnight. Cut into ⅛ in. (4 mm) slices. Then bake on lightly oiled cookie sheet at 375 °F (190 °C) for 6 minutes or until golden brown.

Yield: 30 servings
Exchange, 1 serving: ¼ high-fat meat
Calories, 1 serving: 22
Carbohydrates, 1 serving: 1

Sweets

Sweet Raisin-Bread Pudding

¾ c.	raisins	190 mL
¼ c.	liquid fructose	60 mL
4 c.	fresh white bread cubes	1000 mL
1 qt.	skim milk	1 L
5	eggs, slightly beaten	5
3 T.	granulated sugar replacement	45 mL
2 t.	vanilla extract	10 mL
¼ t.	salt	1 mL
dash	nutmeg	dash

Rinse raisins under cold water and drain. Combine liquid fructose and bread cubes in a saucepan. While stirring, cook over low heat until bread cubes absorb the fructose. Remove from heat and add raisins. Combine milk, eggs, sugar replacement, vanilla, salt, and nutmeg in a bowl. Stir to blend thoroughly. Pour over bread cubes. Stir to mix well. Transfer to baking dish lightly sprayed with oil. Sprinkle with additional nutmeg. Place baking dish in pan of hot water (hot water should be at least 1 in. [2.5 cm] up the sides of the baking dish). Then bake at 350 °F (175 °C) for an hour or until knife inserted in center comes out clean. The liquid fructose makes this pudding taste as if it were made with honey.

Yield: 8 servings
Exchange, 1 serving: ½ starch/bread, ¾ fruit, ½ skim milk, ¾ medium-
fat meat
Calories, 1 serving: 189
Carbohydrates, 1 serving: 24

Cranberry-Nut Cobbler

4 c.	cranberries	1000 mL
1 c.	water	250 mL
½ c.	granulated sugar replacement	125 mL
2 T.	granulated fructose	30 mL
⅓ c.	walnuts, chopped	90 mL
1 T.	grated, fresh orange rind	15 mL
1 T.	low-calorie margarine	15 mL
10 (1 tube)	biscuits, unbaked	10 (1 tube)

Wash and sort cranberries. Combine cranberries, water, sugar replacement, and fructose in a saucepan. Bring to a boil. Add walnuts, orange rind, and margarine. Remove from heat and allow to stand for 5 minutes. Then spoon cranberry mixture into 10 individual baking dishes. Cut slit in the top of each unbaked biscuit. Place biscuit on top of cranberry mixture. Bake at 450 °F (230 °C) for 10 minutes. Then reduce heat to 350 °F (175 °C) and bake 20 minutes longer.

Yield: 10 cobblers
Exchange, 1 cobbler: 1 starch/bread, ½ fat
Calories, 1 cobbler: 118
Carbohydrates, 1 cobbler: 18

Peanut-Butter Chocolate Quickies

⅓ c.	peanut butter	90 mL
⅓ c.	granulated sugar replacement	90 mL
1	egg, slightly beaten	1
1 T.	water	5 mL
¼ t.	vegetable oil	1 mL
1 c.	biscuit mix	250 mL
¼ c.	mini-chocolate chips	60 mL

Cream peanut butter and sugar replacement; then beat in egg, water, and vegetable oil. Add biscuit mix. Stir until well blended. Stir in chocolate chips. Drop by teaspoonfuls onto a lightly greased cookie sheet. Bake at 350 °F (175 °C) for 10 to 12 minutes

Yield: 30 cookies
Exchange, 1 cookie: ½ starch/bread
Calories, 1 cookie: 42
Carbohydrates, 1 cookie: 6

Brazil Nut Pudding

¼ c.	low-calorie margarine	60 mL
¼ c.	granulated sugar replacement	60 mL
¼ c.	granulated fructose	60 mL
1	egg yolk	1
½ c.	grated apple	125 mL
¼ c.	finely cut dates	60 mL
⅓ c.	chopped Brazil nuts	90 mL
¾ c.	all-purpose flour	190 mL
1 t.	baking powder	5 mL
¼ t.	salt	1 mL
½ c.	coffee, very strong	125 mL
1	egg white, stiffly beaten	1

Cream together margarine, sugar replacement, and fructose until fluffy. Add egg yolk, apple, dates, and Brazil nuts. Mix together flour, baking powder, and salt. Add alternately with strong coffee to creamed mixture. Fold in stiffly beaten egg white. Transfer to 2 qt. (2 L) ring mould or tube pan lightly sprayed with oil. Then bake at 350 °F (175 °C) for 40 to 50 minutes or until done.

Yield: 10 servings
Exchange, 1 serving: 1 starch/bread, 1 fat
Calories, 1 serving: 129
Carbohydrates, 1 serving: 15

Chocolate Bread Pudding

2 oz.	unsweetened baking chocolate	60 g
3 c.	skim milk	750 mL
¼ t.	salt	1 mL
¼ c.	granulated brown-sugar replacement	60 mL
2	eggs, separated	2
2 t.	vanilla extract	10 mL
6 slices	dry white bread, cut in cubes	6 slices
2 T.	granulated sugar replacement	30 mL

Heat chocolate and milk in top of double boiler until chocolate is melted. (If you are using the liquid chocolate, stir chocolate and milk together in a bowl.) Add salt. Combine brown-sugar replacement and egg yolks; then beat slightly to blend. Gradually add to chocolate mixture, while constantly stirring. Add vanilla. Combine bread cubes and chocolate mixture. Allow to rest for 15 minutes, stirring occasionally. Transfer to a baking dish lightly sprayed with oil, and then place dish in a pan of hot water. Bake at 350 °F (175 °C) for 30 minutes or until pudding is almost firm. Beat egg whites until foamy; then add sugar replacement—one teaspoonful (5 mL) at a time. Beat until egg whites stand up in points. Lightly pile egg whites about into mounds in border around edge of chocolate pudding. Bake about 8 minutes longer or until egg whites are lightly browned. This pudding is a chocolate lover's dream come true.

Yield: 12 servings
Exchange, 1 serving: ½ starch/bread, ⅔ medium-fat meat
Calories, 1 serving: 109
Carbohydrates, 1 serving: 18

Moist Carrot Ring

1½ c.	granulated sugar replacement	375 mL
1 c.	vegetable oil	250 mL
3 c.	all-purpose flour	750 mL
1 T.	baking powder	15 mL
1½ t.	cinnamon	7 mL
1 t.	baking soda	5 mL
½ t.	nutmeg	2 mL
¼ t.	salt	1 mL
4	eggs	4
2 c.	coarsely grated carrots	500 mL
½ c.	raisins	125 mL
½ c.	chopped walnuts	125 mL

Beat the sugar replacement with the oil. Combine flour, baking powder, cinnamon, baking soda, nutmeg, and salt together in a bowl. Stir to mix. Add alternately with eggs to oil mixture. Stir in carrots, raisins, and walnuts. If dough is very thick, add a small amount of extra water. Transfer to a greased 10 in. (25 cm) tube pan. Then bake at 350 °F (175 °C) for 45 to 60 minutes or until done.

Yield: 25 servings
Exchange, 1 serving: 1 starch/bread, 2 fats
Calories, 1 serving: 182
Carbohydrates, 1 serving: 17

Cornmeal Pudding

½ c.	yellow cornmeal	125 mL
1 qt.	skim milk, hot	1 L
⅔ c.	dietetic maple syrup	180 mL
1 t.	salt	5 mL
2 c.	skim milk	500 mL

While stirring constantly, add cornmeal slowly to the 1 qt. (l L) of hot milk. Continue to stir, cook over low heat until mixture is thick. Add maple syrup and salt. Transfer to greased baking dish. Add the 2 c. (500 mL) of cold milk. Bake at 275 °F (135 °C) for 3 hours.

Yield: 12 servings
Exchange, 1 serving: 1 starch/bread
Calories, 1 serving: 78
Carbohydrates, 1 serving: 14

Date Roll-Ups

1 c.	water	250 mL
½ c.	chopped dates	125 mL
½ c.	low-calorie margarine	125 mL
½ c.	granulated fructose	125 mL
1 T.	hot water	15 mL
1	egg	1
1 t.	vanilla extract	5 mL
2 c.	all-purpose flour	500 mL
½ t.	salt	2 mL
½ t.	baking soda	2 mL

Combine water and dates in a saucepan. While stirring, cook until mixture becomes a purée. (You might want to grind in a blender after dates become soft and then continue cooking.) Mixture must be thick. Allow to cool completely. Then cream together margarine, fructose, and water. Add egg and vanilla. Beat until smooth. Sift flour, salt, and baking soda together. Gradually add flour to creamed mixture. Beat until well blended. Divide into three parts and then roll out to ¼ in. (8 mm) thick. Spread each part with one third of the date mixture, leaving about ¼ in. (8 mm) around the edge. Roll up jelly-roll fashion. Wrap in plastic wrap and refrigerate to thoroughly chill (at least 3 hours). Slice into ¼ in. (8 mm) cookies. Then bake at 375 °F (190 °C) until brown.

Yield: 66 cookies
Exchange, 1 cookie: ⅓ starch/bread
Calories, 1 cookie: 30
Carbohydrates, 1 cookie: 6

Peach-Rice Custard Loaf

29-oz. can	peaches, in their own juice	826-g can
½ c.	granulated sugar replacement	125 mL
2 T.	granulated fructose	30 mL
¼ c.	all-purpose flour	60 mL
¼ t.	salt	1 mL
1½ c.	skim milk	375 mL
2	egg yolks	2
1½ t.	almond extract	7 mL
2 c.	cooked rice	500 mL
1 c.	dry bread crumbs, sifted	250 mL

Thoroughly drain peaches. Set aside. Combine sugar replacement, fructose, flour, and salt in top of a double boiler. Stir in ½ c. (125 mL) of the milk and the egg yolks; then beat well. Add remaining milk and cook for about 20 minutes over simmering water until thickened. Remove from heat, and stir in almond extract. Fold custard mixture into rice. Cover bottom of greased loaf pan with half of the bread crumbs; then pour in a third of the rice custard. Cover with half of the peaches. Repeat layering of one-third custard, remaining peaches, and then remaining third of custard. Sprinkle with remaining bread crumbs. Bake at 350 °F (175 °C) for 40 to 45 minutes. Allow loaf to cool for 15 minutes before unmoulding. Slice to serve.

Yield: 10 servings
Exchange, 1 serving: 1 starch/bread, ½ lean meat, ½ fruit
Calories, 1 serving: 152
Carbohydrates, 1 serving: 22

Devil's Food Pudding

2 c.	all-purpose flour	500 mL
1 t.	baking soda	5 mL
½ t.	salt	2 mL
3 oz.	unsweetened baking chocolate	90 g
½ c.	granulated sugar replacement	125 mL
1½ c.	skim milk	375 mL
½ c.	solid vegetable shortening	125 mL
¼ c.	granulated fructose	60 mL
2 T.	liquid dietetic sweetener	30 mL
2	eggs, beaten	2
1 t.	vanilla extract	5 mL

Sift flour, baking soda, and salt together. Melt chocolate in top of double boiler; then add sugar replacement and ½ c. (125 mL) of the skim milk. Cook until thickened, stirring constantly. Allow to cool. Cream together shortening, fructose, and liquid sweetener until fluffy. Add eggs and beat well. Stir in chocolate mixture. Combine remaining milk and vanilla. Add alternately with the flour to the chocolate mixture. Transfer into a greased and paper-lined 10 in. (25 cm) tube pan. Then bake at 350 °F (175 °C) for 65 to 75 minutes or until done.

Yield: 25 servings
Exchange, 1 serving: ⅔ starch/bread, 1 fat
Calories, 1 serving: 103
Carbohydrates, 1 serving: 9

Buttermilk-Lemon Pound Cake

1 c.	low-calorie margarine, softened	250 mL
½ c.	granulated fructose	125 mL
5	eggs	5
1½ t.	unsweetened lemon-drink mix	7 mL
1 t.	vanilla extract	5 mL
3 c.	sifted all-purpose flour	750 mL
1 t.	baking soda	5 mL
1 t.	baking powder	5 mL
¾ c.	buttermilk	190 mL

The mixing is very important in this recipe; make sure you beat the batter well. Cream the margarine first. Then slowly add the fructose and beat until well blended and fluffy. Beat in eggs, one at a time. Beat 2 minutes after each addition. Beat in lemon-drink mix and vanilla. (If you are using pre-sifted flour, you must sift it again and measure it before sifting it with the baking soda and baking powder.) Sift flour, baking soda, and baking powder together. Add alternately with buttermilk to creamed mixture, beating continuously. Spray a Bundt pan with vegetable oil. Now transfer cake dough to pan and level it out. Bake at 350 °F (175 °C) for 45 to 60 minutes or until toothpick inserted in center comes out clean.

Yield: 25 servings
Exchange, 1 serving: ¾ starch/bread, 1½ fat
Calories, 1 serving: 139
Carbohydrates, 1 serving: 13

Rhubarb Crisp

½ c.	granulated sugar replacement	125 mL
½ c.	granulated fructose	125 mL
½ c.	low-calorie margarine	125 mL
2	eggs	2
1 t.	nutmeg	5 mL
1 t.	vanilla extract	5 mL
2 c.	bread cubes, toasted	500 mL
4 c.	cornflakes	1000 mL
4 c.	diced fresh rhubarb	1000 mL

Combine sugar replacement and fructose in a bowl. Stir to mix. Thoroughly blend together the margarine and half of the sweetener mixture. Add eggs and beat well. Next, stir in nutmeg, vanilla, toasted bread cubes, and cornflakes. Spread half of the mixture in the bottom of two 9 in. (23-cm)-square greased baking pans. Then arrange rhubarb evenly over the top. Sprinkle with remaining sweetener mixture, and cover with remaining cornflakes mixture. Bake at 375 °F (190 °C) for 40 to 45 minutes or until rhubarb is tender. This is a perfect afternoon snack.

Yield: 18 servings
Exchange, 1 serving: 1 starch/bread, 1 fat
Calories, 1 serving: 126
Carbohydrates, 1 serving: 13

Vanilla Wafers

⅓ c.	low-calorie margarine	90 mL
¼ c.	granulated sugar replacement	60 mL
¼ c.	granulated fructose	60 mL
1	egg, slightly beaten	1
2 T.	water	30 mL
1 t.	vanilla extract	5 mL
2 c.	all-purpose flour	500 mL
2 t.	baking powder	10 mL
½ t.	salt	2 mL

Cream together margarine, sugar replacement, and fructose in a mixing bowl. Add egg, water, and vanilla. Beat until well blended. Combine flour, baking powder, and salt in a sifter. Sift to thoroughly mix. Beat into creamed mixture. Form into two 8 in. (20 cm) × 1 in (2.5 cm) rolls. Wrap each roll in plastic wrap. Chill thoroughly. Cut into ⅛ in. (4 mm) slices. Place on a cookie sheet sprayed lightly with vegetable oil. Then bake at 375 °F (190 °C) for 8 to 10 minutes. You'll be using this basic recipe in some of the cookie recipes that follow.

Yield: 126 cookies
Exchange, 3 cookies: ⅓ starch/bread
Calories, 3 cookies: 33
Carbohydrates, 3 cookies: 5

Orange Cookies

1 recipe	Vanilla Wafers, unbaked	1 recipe
1 T.	finely chopped fresh orange zest	15 mL
1 t.	orange flavoring	5 mL
1 t.	unsweetened orange-drink mix	5 mL

Prepare wafers as directed in previous recipe, adding the orange zest, orange flavoring, and orange-drink mix along with the flour mixture. Then bake at 375 °F (190 °C) for 8 to 10 minutes.

Yield: 126 cookies
Exchange, 3 cookies: ⅓ starch/bread
Calories, 3 cookies: 34
Carbohydrates, 3 cookies: 5

Nut Wafers

1 recipe	Vanilla Wafers, unbaked	1 recipe
⅓ c.	powdered pecans	90 mL

Prepare wafers as directed in Vanilla Wafers recipe, adding powdered pecans along with the flour mixture. Then bake at 375 °F (190 °C) for 8 to 10 minutes.

Yield: 126 cookies
Exchange, 3 cookies: ⅓ starch/bread, ¼ fat
Calories, 3 cookies: 45
Carbohydrates, 3 cookies: 6

Spiced-Apple Yogurt Cake

⅓ c.	slivered almonds, lightly toasted	90 mL
1 c.	low-calorie margarine, softened	250 mL
½ c.	granulated sugar replacement	125 mL
5	eggs	5
1 t.	apple flavoring	5 mL
1 t.	vanilla extract	5 mL
3 c.	all-purpose flour	750 mL
1 t.	baking soda	5 mL
1 t.	baking powder	5 mL
8 oz.	low-calorie apple-spice yogurt	240 g

Grease a 10 in. (25 cm) tube pan. Sprinkle with toasted slivered almonds. Cream together margarine and sugar replacement until fluffy. Add eggs, one at a time, beating well after each addition. Add apple flavoring and vanilla. Sift flour, baking soda, and baking powder together. Add alternately with yogurt to creamed mixture. Beat well after each addition. Transfer to the prepared tube pan. Then bake at 350 °F (175 °C) for 45 to 60 minutes.

Yield: 25 servings
Exchange, 1 serving: 1 starch/bread, 1½ fat
Calories, 1 serving: 157
Carbohydrates, 1 serving: 15

Prune Betty

4 c.	bread cubes, toasted	1000 mL
1½ c.	sliced cooked prunes	375 mL
1½ c.	chopped apples	375 mL
1 c.	prune liquid	250 mL
¾ c.	water	190 mL
½ c.	granulated sugar replacement	125 mL
½ t.	salt	2 mL
½ t.	cinnamon	2 mL
2 T.	low-calorie margarine, melted	30 mL

Place half of the toasted bread cubes in a 2 qt. (2 L) baking dish lightly sprayed with vegetable oil. Add prunes and apples in layers. Top with remaining bread cubes. Combine prune liquid, water, sugar replacement, salt, cinnamon, and margarine in a saucepan. Bring to a boil. Reduce heat and cook for 3 minutes. Pour hot liquid over bread cubes. Then cover and bake at 375 °F (190 °C) for 60 minutes. This is a fast and very easy snack to prepare.

Yield: 12 servings
Exchange, 1 serving: ⅓ starch/bread, ⅔ fruit
Calories, 1 serving: 69
Carbohydrates, 1 serving: 16

Peanut-Butter Cookies

½ c.	creamy peanut butter	125 mL
2 T.	granulated brown-sugar replacement	30 mL
2 T.	granulated sugar replacement	30 mL
1	egg, slightly beaten	1
3 T.	water	45 mL
1 c.	biscuit mix	250 mL

Cream together peanut butter and both sugar replacements; then beat in egg and water. Add biscuit mix. Stir until well blended. Drop by teaspoonfuls onto a lightly greased cookie sheet. Bake at 350 °F (175 °C) for 10 to 12 minutes.

Yield: 30 cookies
Exchange, 1 cookie: ½ starch/bread
Calories, 1 cookie: 45
Carbohydrates, 1 cookie: 6

Frozen Treats

Creamy Chocolate Ice

13-oz. pkg.	sugar-free instant chocolate pudding mix	377-g pkg.
1 qt.	2% low-fat milk	1 L

Combine pudding mix and milk in large bowl. With a wire whisk, rotary beater, or electric mixer on low speed, blend thoroughly. Pour into ice-cream maker. Freeze as directed by manufacturer. Then serve immediately or pack in freezer container for later use.

Yield: 8 servings
Exchange, 1 serving: 1 low-fat milk
Calories, 1 serving: 82
Carbohydrates, 1 serving: 12

Pistachio Cream

12-oz. can	evaporated skim milk	354-g can
13-oz. package	sugar-free instant pistachio pudding mix	377-g package

Chill evaporated milk thoroughly. Pour into 1 qt. (1 L) measuring cup. Add enough cold water to make 3 c. (750 mL) liquid. Next, add pudding mix. With a wire whisk, beat until well blended. Pour into ice-cream maker. Freeze as directed by manufacturer. Serve immediately or pack in freezer container for later use.

Yield: 6 servings
Exchange, 1 serving: 1 starch/bread
Calories, 1 serving: 73
Carbohydrates, 1 serving: 11

Strawberry Delight

13-oz. package	sugar-free instant vanilla pudding mix	377-g package
3 c.	skim milk	750 mL
1 T.	nondairy whipped-topping mix	15 mL
1 c.	sliced strawberries	250 mL
6 whole	strawberries	6 whole

Combine pudding mix, skim milk, and nondairy whipped-topping mix in bowl. With a wire whisk, hand beater, or electric mixer at low speed, blend to thoroughly mix. Pour into ice-cream maker. Freeze as directed by manufacturer. Approximately halfway through freezing, add the sliced strawberries. Continue freezing. To serve: Top each dish with one whole strawberry.

Yield: 6 servings
Exchange, 1 serving: 1 skim milk
Calories, 1 serving: 80
Carbohydrates, 1 serving: 14

Eggnog Ice Cream

2	eggs, separated	2
3 env.	aspartame low-calorie sweetener	3 env.
2 T.	brandy flavoring	30 mL
2 T.	rum flavoring	30 mL
1 c.	skim milk, hot	250 mL
1 env.	nondairy whipped-topping mix	1 env.
½ c.	cold water	125 mL

Beat egg yolks until thick and lemon colored. Beat in sweetener, brandy flavoring, rum flavoring, and hot skim milk. Chill thoroughly. Beat egg whites until stiff. Combine nondairy whipped-topping mix and cold water in a bowl. Beat into soft peaks. Fold egg-yolk mixture into stiffly beaten egg whites, and then into whipped topping. Pour into ice-cream maker. Freeze as directed by manufacturer. Serve immediately or pack in freezer container for later use.

Yield: 8 servings
Exchange, 1 serving: ⅓ fruit, ¼ medium-fat meat
Calories, 1 serving: 63
Carbohydrates, 1 serving: 5

Mandarin Crown

13-oz. pkg.	sugar-free instant vanilla pudding mix	377-g pkg.
2 c.	skim milk	500 mL
2	egg whites	2
½ c.	evaporated skim milk, chilled icy cold	125 mL
½ t.	vanilla extract	3 mL
1 T.	lemon juice	30 mL
11-oz. can	mandarin orange sections, drained	319-g can

Combine pudding mix and skim milk in large mixing bowl. Stir just to blend. Beat egg whites until soft peaks form. Add vanilla and lemon juice. Beat until fluffy. Fold into pudding mixture. Beat evaporated skim milk until soft peaks form. Fold into pudding mixture. Fold in mandarin orange sections. Then turn into ice-cream maker. Freeze as directed by manufacturer. Serve immediately or pack in freezer container for later use.

Yield: 8 servings
Exchange, 1 serving: ⅔ skim milk, ¼ fruit
Calories, 1 serving: 70
Carbohydrates, 1 serving: 13

Strawberry-Rum Freeze

3 c.	skim milk	750 mL
2 T.	nondairy whipped-topping mix	30 mL
1 T.	rum flavoring	15 mL
½ c.	crushed strawberries	125 mL
1 t.	strawberry flavoring	5 mL
6 whole	strawberries	6 whole

Combine milk, whipped-topping mix, and rum flavoring in a bowl. With a rotary beater or electric mixer, beat until blended. Pour into ice-cream maker. Freeze to desired consistency, following manufacturer's directions. Halfway through freezing, add crushed strawberries and strawberry flavoring. Continue freezing. Serve in stemmed glasses, and top with strawberries. This is similar to a strawberry daiquiri.

Yield: 6 servings
Exchange, 1 serving: ¾ skim milk
Calories, 1 serving: 54
Carbohydrates, 1 serving: 8

Vanilla Pudding Ice

| 13-oz. pkg. | sugar-free instant vanilla pudding mix | 377-g pkg. |
| 1 qt. | 2% milk | 1 L |

Combine pudding mix and milk in large bowl. With a wire whisk, rotary beater, or electric mixer on low speed, blend thoroughly. Pour into ice-cream maker. Freeze as directed by manufacturer. Then serve immediately or pack in freezer container for later use.

Yield: 8 servings
Exchange, 1 serving: 1 low-fat milk
Calories, 1 serving: 80
Carbohydrates, 1 serving: 10

Prune Ice Cream

1 t.	unflavored gelatin	5 mL
1 T.	cold water	15 mL
2 c.	prunes	500 mL
1 c.	skim milk	250 mL
4	eggs, beaten	4
1 T.	vanilla extract	15 mL
¼ t.	salt	1 mL
1 env.	nondairy whipped-topping mix	1 env.
½ c.	cold water	125 mL

Soften gelatin in the 1 T. (15 mL) of cold water for 5 minutes. Wash prunes in hot water, cut out pit, and place in blender or food processor. Add ½ c. (125 mL) of the skim milk. Blend thoroughly until prunes are in small pieces. Combine remaining skim milk, prune mixture, and gelatin in a saucepan. Bring to boiling. Slowly pour hot mixture over beaten eggs, stirring constantly. Add vanilla and salt. Chill thoroughly. Combine nondairy whipped-topping mix and the ½ c. (125 mL) of cold water in a bowl. Beat to soft peaks. Then fold cooled prune mixture into whipped topping. Pour into ice-cream maker. Freeze as directed by manufacturer. Serve immediately or pack in freezer container for later use.

Yield: 12 servings
Exchange, 1 serving: ⅔ fruit, ⅓ medium-fat meat
Calories, 1 serving: 76
Carbohydrates, 1 serving: 10

Blueberry Supreme Cream

3 env.	aspartame low-calorie sweetener	3 env.
1 qt.	buttermilk	1 L
1½ c.	frozen blueberries (no added sugar)	375 mL

Stir sweetener into buttermilk until completely dissolved. Pour into ice-cream maker. Freeze as directed by manufacturer. Halfway through freezing, add blueberries. Continue freezing. Serve immediately or pack in freezer containers for later use.

Yield: 6 servings
Exchange, 1 serving: ½ low-fat milk, ½ fruit
Calories, 1 serving: 89
Carbohydrates, 1 serving: 13

Icy Mint

3 c.	2% low-fat milk	750 mL
1 T.	wintergreen flavoring	30 mL
3 drops	green food coloring	3 drops

Combine all ingredients in a bowl. Stir to mix. Pour into ice-cream maker. Freeze to desired consistency, following manufacturer's directions. If this is served soft, it will be similiar to a Grasshopper.

Yield: 4 servings
Exchange, 1 serving: ¾ skim milk
Calories, 1 serving: 67
Carbohydrates, 1 serving: 9

Pina Colada Cooler

2 c.	unsweetened pineapple juice	500 mL
¼ c.	unsweetened flaked coconut	60 mL
¼ c.	cold water	60 mL
2 t.	rum flavoring	10 mL

Combine all ingredients in a bowl. Stir to mix. Pour into ice-cream maker. Freeze to desired consistency.

Yield: 4 servings
Exchange, 1 serving: 1 fruit, ½ fat
Calories, 1 serving: 87
Carbohydrates, 1 serving: 16

Three-Fruit Sherbet

1	banana, very ripe	1
1 c.	orange juice	250 mL
13-oz. can	pineapple chunks in their own juice	384-g can
1 env.	nondairy whipped topping mix	1 env.

Combine all ingredients in a food processor or electric mixer. Beat until thoroughly blended and frothy. Pour into ice-cream maker. Freeze as directed by manufacturer. Then serve immediately or pack in freezer container for later use.

Yield: 8 servings
Exchange, 1 serving: 1½ fruit
Calories, 1 serving: 90
Carbohydrates, 1 serving: 19

Pineapple-Rum Delight

2 c.	2% low-fat milk	500 mL
2 t.	rum flavoring	10 mL
⅓ c.	crushed pineapple, in its own juice	90 mL

Combine milk and rum flavoring in a bowl. Stir to mix. Pour into ice-cream maker. Freeze to desired consistency. Halfway through freezing, add crushed pineapple. Then continue freezing.

Yield: 3 servings
Exchange, 1 serving: ¾ skim milk
Calories, 1 serving: 71
Carbohydrates, 1 serving: 11

Cooling Stinger

3 c.	skim milk	750 mL
2 T.	brandy flavoring	30 mL
1 T.	wintergreen flavoring	15 mL

Combine all ingredients in a bowl. Stir to mix. Pour into ice-cream maker. Freeze to desired consistency.

Yield: 4 servings
Exchange, 1 serving: ¾ skim milk
Calories, 1 serving: 68
Carbohydrates, 1 serving: 9

Kids' Stuff

Ole Banana Train

1	banana	1
2 T.	peanut butter	30 mL

Peel banana. With a table knife, cut the banana into round slices. Spread each slice with a small amount of peanut butter. Press the banana slices with the peanut butter in between together. You just made a Banana Train. Eat.

Yield: 1 serving
Exchange, 1 serving: 1⅔ fruit, 3 fats
Calories, 1 serving: 235
Carbohydrates, 1 serving: 26

Red Fruit Rouges

1 qt.	strawberries, hulled	1 L
10-oz. pkg.	frozen raspberries (no added sugar), partially thawed	280-g pkg.
1 c.	prepared nondairy whipped topping	250 mL

Arrange strawberries in a pyramid on a chilled serving dish. Drain excess liquid from partially thawed raspberries. Break raspberries into large chunks and place in blender. Process at high speed into a thick purée. Then pour over strawberries. Serve with prepared nondairy whipped topping.

Yield: 10 servings
Exchange, 1 serving: 1 fruit
Calories, 1 serving: 56
Carbohydrates, 1 serving: 12

Banana Split

1	banana	1
½ t.	lemon juice	2 mL
4 leaves	lettuce	4 leaves
¼ c.	fresh grapefruit sections	60 mL
¼ c.	seedless purple grapes	60 mL
4	fresh orange sections	4

Peel banana and cut in half crosswise. Cut each half banana into four sections lengthwise. Sprinkle with lemon juice. Place two sections of banana on a leaf of lettuce on four small plates. Evenly distribute the grapefruit between the banana slices. Distribute the purple grapes evenly between the plates. Next, top each plate with an orange slice. Serve immediately, or cover with plastic wrap and keep refrigerated until serving time.

Yield: 4 servings
Exchange, 1 serving: ⅔ fruit
Calories, 1 serving: 41
Carbohydrates, 1 serving: 10

Dried-Fruit Medley

½ c.	dried apples	125 mL
½ c.	dried apricots	125 mL
⅓ c.	dried peaches	90 mL
⅓ c.	dried pears	90 mL
¼ c.	lemon juice	60 mL
3 env.	Equal low-calorie sweetener	3 env.

Combine all dried fruits in saucepan. Cover with water; then cover saucepan and simmer until fruits are almost tender. Add lemon juice. Continue cooking until fruits are tender. Add extra water if needed. Cool to room temperature. Stir in Equal. Chill thoroughly. If stored in a tightly covered refrigerator bowl, this should keep at least 2 weeks. Make it at least a day before to allow the flavors to mingle.

Yield: 12 servings
Exchange, 1 serving: ⅔ fruit
Calories, 1 serving: 45
Carbohydrates, 1 serving: 11

Golden Apricot Mould

2 (16 oz.) cans	apricot halves, in their own juice	2 (454 g) cans
¼ c.	vinegar	60 mL
1 t.	whole cloves	5 mL
4 inches	cinnamon stick	10 cm
1 env.	dietetic orange-flavor gelatin	1 env.

Shiny cups of orange gelatin with apricot halves. . . . First, drain juice from apricots into saucepan. Then add vinegar, cloves, and cinnamon stick, and bring to a boil. Add apricots; then reduce heat and simmer for 5 minutes. With a slotted spoon, remove apricots to 10 individual moulds. Strain liquid and measure, and then add enough hot water to make 2 cups (500 mL). Add gelatin and stir to completely dissolve. (If gelatin does not dissolve, return liquid to saucepan and cook, while stirring, until gelatin dissolves.) Pour gelatin mixture over apricots in moulds. Chill until firm. Turn out onto chilled platter or plates.

Yield: 10 servings
Exchange, 1 serving: ⅔ fruit
Calories, 1 serving: 43
Carbohydrates, 1 serving: 11

Spicy Cereal Mix

3 c.	bite-size corn cereal biscuits	750 mL
3 c.	bite-size wheat cereal biscuits	750 mL
3 c.	bite-size rice cereal biscuits	750 mL
1 c.	salted peanuts	250 mL
⅓ c.	low-calorie margarine, melted	90 mL
1 t.	chili powder	5 mL
1 T.	Mexican spices	15 mL

Combine all ingredients in a large bowl. Toss to completely blend. Turn out onto a cookie sheet. Bake at 250 °F (125 °C) for 45 minutes. While stirring, mix cereal every 15 minutes. Turn out onto paper towelling to cool.

Yield: 20 servings
Exchange, 1 serving: 1 starch/bread, 1 fat
Calories, 1 serving: 132
Carbohydrates, 1 serving: 14

Stuffed Apple

1	apple	1
¼ c.	cornflakes	60 mL
2 T.	chunky peanut butter	30 mL

With a spoon, cut around the stem of the apple. Throw away the core and stem. Dig out and remove the inside of the apple. In a bowl, combine the apple pieces from the inside of the apple, the cornflakes, and peanut butter. Mix together. Fill the hole in the apple with the mixture. Eat.

Yield: 1 serving
Exchange, 1 serving: 1 fruit, ⅓ starch/bread, 3 fats
Calories, 1 serving: 273
Carbohydrates, 1 serving: 26

Mountain Salad

1	pineapple ring, in its own juice	1
1 leaf	iceberg lettuce	1 leaf
⅓ c.	low-calorie cottage cheese	90 mL
1 env.	aspartame low-calorie sweetener	1 env.
dash	nutmeg	dash

Drain the pineapple ring. Place lettuce leaf on chilled plate. Top with pineapple ring. Mix cottage cheese and sweetener together. Mound the cottage cheese on top of pineapple ring. Then sprinkle with nutmeg.

Yield: 1 serving
Exchange, 1 serving: 1 fruit, ⅔ skim milk
Calories, 1 serving: 115
Carbohydrates, 1 serving: 17

Pink Pears

| 16-oz. can | pear halves, in their own juice | 454-mL can |
| 4 drops | red food coloring | 4 drops |

Drain juice from pears into a glass bowl. Add red food coloring and stir to blend. Add pears, making sure they are completely immersed in the liquid. Cover and refrigerate at least one day to chill and gain the pink color. With a slotted spoon, remove pear halves to four chilled lettuce-trimmed plates. Optional: Place a mint sprig in the center cavity of each pear half. Color usually adds life to a table.

Yield: 4 servings
Exchange, 1 serving: 1 fruit
Calories, 1 serving: 60
Carbohydrates, 1 serving: 15

Prairie Greens

½ lb.	spinach, rinsed	250 g
2 t.	low-calorie margarine	10 mL
¼ t.	salt	1 mL
dash each	oregano, basil, thyme	dash each

Place spinach in a saucepan with ¼ c. (60 mL) of water. Cover and cook over low heat until spinach wilts. Remove lid and cook until liquid evaporates. Add remaining ingredients. Then toss lightly to mix.

Yield: 1 serving
Exchange, 1 serving: 1 fat
Calories, 1 serving: 35
Carbohydrates, 1 serving: negligible

Stuffed Celery

1	celery stalk, rinsed	1
¼ c.	low-calorie cottage cheese	60 mL
1 t.	Mexican spice mix	5 mL

Remove threadlike fibers from back of celery stalk by loosening the fiber piece with your finger or a table knife. Pull the thread down the stalk. Combine cottage cheese and spice mix in a small bowl. Stir to blend. Then fill cavity of celery stalk with cottage-cheese mixture.

Yield: 1 serving
Exchange, 1 serving: ½ skim milk
Calories, 1 serving: 41
Carbohydrates, 1 serving: 2

Cucumber Cubes

2 T.	ketchup	30 mL
½ t.	Worcestershire sauce	2 mL
¼ t.	horseradish	1 mL
	black pepper	
1 large	cucumber	1 large

Combine ketchup, Worcestershire sauce, horseradish, and pepper in small bowl. Stir to blend. Peel cucumber and then cut into ¼ in. (8 mm) cubes. Place cucumber cubes in bowl. Cover with sauce.

Yield: 1 serving
Exchange, 1 serving: negligible
Calories, 1 serving: negligible
Carbohydrates, 1 serving: negligible

Peanut-Butter Balls

| ½ c. | chunky peanut butter | 125 mL |
| 1 c. | wheat germ | 250 mL |

Combine ingredients in a bowl. Mix together thoroughly. With your hands, roll small amounts of the mixture into small balls. Place on a plate. Refrigerate until firm.

Yield: 10 servings
Exchange, 1 serving: ⅓ starch/bread, 1½ fats
Calories, 1 serving: 94
Carbohydrates, 1 serving: 5

Worms

| ½ c. | chunky peanut butter | 125 mL |
| ½ c. | nonfat dry milk powder | 125 mL |

Combine ingredients in a bowl. Mix together thoroughly. Divide the dough into five equal parts. With your hands, shape the dough into 10 "worms." Place on a plate or wrap in waxed paper. Then refrigerate until firm.

Yield: 10 servings
Exchange, 1 serving: ⅙ skim milk, 1½ fats
Calories, 1 serving: 81
Carbohydrates, 1 serving: 2

Beef Jerky

2 lbs   flank steak   1 kg
         soy sauce

Trim all fat and gristle from meat. Cut into ⅛ in. (4 mm) slices. Lay flat in a dish or marinade container. Cover with soy sauce. Allow to marinade at least 2 days. Remove from soy sauce and dry slightly. Place beef slices on a cookie sheet. Sprinkle with black pepper, if desired. Bake at 250 °F (125 °C) for about 8 hours. Turn meat several times during baking. Or place directly on rack in oven, with a pan under beef to collect any drippings. This can also be done in a smoker, according to manufacturer's directions.

Yield: 22 servings
Exchange, 1 serving: 1 lean meat
Calories, 1 serving: 57
Carbohydrates, 1 serving: negligible

Orangey Cooler

2 c.   orange juice   500 mL
1 t.   low-calorie orange-flavored drink mix   5 mL

Dissolve drink mix in orange juice. Pour orange mixture into ice-cream maker. Freeze according to manufacturer's directions. Serve immediately, or pack and freeze for later use.

Yield: 2 servings
Exchange, 1 serving: 2 fruit
Calories, 1 serving: 120
Carbohydrates, 1 serving: 29

Easy Chocolate Freeze

1 qt.   low-fat chocolate milk   1 L

Pour chocolate milk into ice-cream maker. Freeze according to manufacturer's directions. Serve immediately, or pack and freeze for later use.

Yield: 6 servings
Exchange, 1 serving: 1 low-fat milk
Calories, 1 serving: 106
Carbohydrates, 1 serving: 13

Nut and Fruit Mix

½ c. each   unsalted pumpkin seeds   125 mL
               walnut halves
               peanuts
               pecans
               unsweetened flaked coconut
               raisins
               diced dried apricots
               diced dried apples

Mix together and store in air-tight container or refrigerate. This dish is easy to make and easy to carry.

Yield: 16 servings
Exchange, 1 serving: ½ fruit, 2 fats
Calories, 1 serving: 121
Carbohydrates, 1 serving: 11

Cran-Orange-Banana Drink

1 c.   low-calorie cranberry-juice cocktail   250 mL
1 c.   orange juice   250 mL
1   banana, sliced   1

Combine ingredients in a blender. Blend on HIGH until thoroughly mixed. Pour into two glasses.

Yield: 2 servings
Exchange, 1 serving: 2 fruit
Calories, 1 serving: 119
Carbohydrates, 1 serving: 29

Rich Apple Milk

1 c.   skim milk   250 mL
½ c.   apple juice   125 mL
⅓ c.   vanilla ice milk   90 mL

Combine ingredients in a blender. Blend thoroughly. Pour into tall glass.

Yield: 1 serving
Exchange, 1 serving: 1⅔ skim milk, ¾ fruit
Calories, 1 serving: 195
Carbohydrates, 1 serving: 21

Almost-Chocolate Shake

1 c.	skim milk	250 mL
2 T.	sugar-free instant chocolate-fudge pudding mix	30 mL

Combine milk and pudding mix in blender. Blend on HIGH until smooth. Pour into glass. If you want it thicker, place in freezer until crystals form on side of container. Blend again.

Yield: 1 serving
Exchange, 1 serving: 1 low-fat milk
Calories, 1 serving: 120
Carbohydrates, 1 serving: 16

Orange-Vanilla Cream

1 c.	skim milk	250 mL
2 t.	aspartame-sweetened orange-drink mix	10 mL
3 T.	prepared nondairy whipped topping	45 mL

Combine milk and orange-drink mix in glass. Stir to dissolve mix. Top with nondairy whipped topping. Stir to blend slightly.

Yield: 1 serving
Exchange, 1 serving: 1 skim milk
Calories, 1 serving: 100
Carbohydrates, 1 serving: 14

Peach Cream

1 c.	frozen peach slices	250 mL
½ c.	skim milk	125 mL
2 T.	low-calorie vanilla yogurt	30 mL
¼ t.	almond extract	1 mL

Combine ingredients in a blender. Blend on HIGH until smooth. Pour into a tall glass.

Yield: 1 serving
Exchange, 1 serving: 1 skim milk, ⅔ fruit
Calories, 1 serving: 135
Carbohydrates, 1 serving: 21

Hot Tomato Fingers

1 c.	finely chopped cooked ham	250 mL
½ c.	shredded cheese	125 mL
1 t.	horseradish	5 mL
1 t.	prepared mustard	5 mL
½ c.	condensed tomato soup	125 mL
6 slices	low-calorie white bread	6 slices

Combine ham, cheese, horseradish, mustard, and tomato soup in a bowl. Stir to mix. Trim crusts from bread slices. Cut each slice into three finger pieces. Spread the ham mixture evenly on all 18 bread fingers. Place bread fingers on a cookie sheet. Then place under a broiler for 3 to 4 minutes or until hot.

Yield: 18 servings
Exchange, 1 serving: $1/_5$ starch/bread, ½ high-fat meat
Calories, 1 serving: 64
Carbohydrates, 1 serving: 3

Vegetable Beef Soup

½ c.	all-purpose flour	125 mL
½ t.	salt	2 mL
⅛ t.	black pepper	½ mL
1 lb.	lean beef, cubed	500 g
2 T.	vegetable oil	30 mL
2 qt.	water	2 L
2 c.	chopped tomatoes (peeled and seeded)	500 mL
2 c.	diced potatoes	500 mL
1 c.	sliced celery	250 mL
½ c.	sliced carrots	125 mL
½ c.	chopped onion	125 mL

Assemble all the ingredients and then start making this *real* soup. It's much more fun eating creations you have made yourself. Now place flour, salt, and pepper in a plastic bag. Add beef cubes in small batches, and shake to coat the cubes with flour. Place the flour-coated cubes on a plate. Heat oil in a large 6 qt. (6 L) soup pot. Add floured beef cubes. While stirring, fry over medium heat until browned. Add remaining ingredients to soup pot. Bring to a boil. Reduce heat, cover, and simmer for 2 to 3 hours or until meat is tender. If needed, add extra salt and pepper to taste.

Yield: 8 servings
Exchange, 1 serving: 1 medium-fat meat, ¾ starch/bread, ¾ vegetable
Calories, 1 serving: 159
Carbohydrates, 1 serving: 14

Fresh Cream of Tomato Soup

2½ c.	chopped tomatoes (peeled and seeded)	625 mL
⅓ c.	chopped onion	90 mL
2 T.	granulated sugar replacement	30 mL
1 t.	salt	5 mL
1 small	bay leaf	1 small
1 T.	low-calorie margarine, melted	15 mL
3 T.	all-purpose flour	45 mL
⅓ c.	cold water	90 mL
2 c.	cold skim milk	500 mL

Combine tomatoes, onion, sugar replacement, salt, and bay leaf in a 2 qt. (2 L) saucepan. Bring to simmering over medium heat. Simmer for 5 minutes. Remove bay leaf. Strain tomato soup, forcing pulp of tomato through sieve. Return sieved tomatoes to saucepan. Stir in melted margarine. Combine flour and cold water in a shaker bottle or bowl. Shake or stir to blend thoroughly. Now slowly pour flour mixture into tomato soup. Return to heat. While stirring constantly, bring mixture to boiling; then cook for 2 minutes. Remove from heat and cool slightly. Now slowly add milk. Stir and reheat, without boiling. Serve hot.

Yield: 6 servings
Exchange, 1 serving: 2 vegetable, ½ fat
Calories, 1 serving: 72
Carbohydrates, 1 serving: 10

Pizza Soup

10-oz. can	tomato soup	304-g can
1 c.	water	250 mL
¼ lb.	lean ground beef, cooked	250 g
3	mushrooms, thinly sliced	3
3 T.	finely chopped onions	45 mL
1 clove	garlic, minced	1 clove
1 t.	oregano	5 mL
¼ c.	shredded mozzarella cheese	60 mL

Combine soup and water in a saucepan. Stir to blend. Add beef, mushrooms, onions, garlic, and oregano. Bring to a boil; then reduce heat and simmer for about 5 minutes or until onions are tender. Stir in cheese. Continue stirring until cheese is slightly melted. Ladle into four bowls. This is like pizza, without the crust.

Yield: 4 servings
Exchange, 1 serving: 2 vegetable, 1 medium-fat meat
Calories, 1 serving: 125
Carbohydrates, 1 serving: 10

Cream-Peanut-Cheese Sandwiches

3-oz. pkg.	cream cheese, softened	90-g pkg.
½ c.	finely chopped fresh parsely	125 mL
⅓ c.	finely chopped salted peanuts	90 mL
2 t.	skim milk	10 mL
½ t.	lemon juice	2 mL
12 slices	low-calorie white bread	12 slices

Cream the cheese until soft. Beat in parsley, peanuts, skim milk, and lemon juice until well blended and mixture is creamy. Trim crusts from bread. Spread creamed mixture thinly on each slice of bread. Then cut bread into squares. Optional: Mixture may be piped on the bread squares with a pastry tube.

Yield: 48 servings
Exchange, 1 serving: ¼ starch/bread, ⅓ fat
Calories, 1 serving: 32
Carbohydrates, 1 serving: 4

Summer Surprise Soup

½ lb.	mushrooms	250 g
2 c.	hot water	500 mL
2 cubes	chicken bouillon	2 cubes
1 env.	unflavored gelatin	1 env.
½ c.	cold water	125 mL
¼ t.	black pepper	1 mL
8 T.	low-calorie plain yogurt	120 mL
2 t.	finely chopped chives or onion	10 mL

Rinse and slice mushrooms. Combine the 2 c. (500 mL) hot water and chicken bouillon cubes in a saucepan. Heat until cubes are dissolved. Add mushrooms; then cover and simmer for 30 minutes. Sprinkle gelatin over the ½ c. (125 mL) cold water and allow to soften. Stir into soup. Add pepper. Remove from heat. Ladle into four soup bowls. Chill until firm. Top each bowl with 2 T. (30 mL) of plain yogurt; then sprinkle with ½ t. (2 mL) of chives. Serve.

Yield: 4 servings
Exchange, 1 serving: ⅓ skim milk
Calories, 1 serving: 35
Carbohydrates, 1 serving: 3

Peanut-Butter Perfect

2	eggs, slightly beaten	2
1½ c.	skim milk	375 mL
⅓ c.	creamy peanut butter	90 mL
6 slices	low-calorie white bread, toasted	6 slices

Combine eggs, milk, and peanut butter in the top of a double boiler. While stirring, cook mixture over simmering water for 12 to 15 minutes or until rich, thick, and creamy. Pour over toast. This is a fun sandwich to make and to eat.

Yield: 6 servings
Exchange, 1 serving: ½ starch/bread, ½ skim milk, 2 fats
Carbohydrates, 1 serving: 13

Peanut-Butter Banana Stick-and-Dip Sandwiches

¼ c.	peanut butter	60 mL
½	banana, mashed	½
6	hard breadsticks	6

My daughter created the name "stick-and-dip sandwiches" because you use a breadstick with the filling instead of spreading it on a piece of bread. First, combine peanut butter and banana in a bowl. Then stir to blend. To eat: Dip the breadstick into the mixture.

Yield: 6 servings
Exchange, 1 serving: ½ starch/bread, 1½ fat
Calories, 1 serving: 131
Carbohydrates, 1 serving: 7

Ham-and-Chicken Stick-and-Dip Sandwiches

¼ c.	condensed cream of mushroom soup	60 mL
¼ c.	finely chopped cooked ham	60 mL
¼ c.	finely chopped cooked chicken	60 mL
1 T.	finely chopped parsley	15 mL
8	hard breadsticks	8

Combine soup, ham, chicken, and parsley in a bowl. Stir to blend. To eat: Dip the breadstick into the mixture.

Yield: 8 servings
Exchange, 1 serving: ⅔ medium-fat meat, ½ starch/bread
Calories, 1 serving: 95
Carbohydrates, 1 serving: 7

Child's Play Egg

2 t.	low-calorie margarine	10 mL
¼ c.	frozen hash-brown potatoes, partially thawed	60 mL
1 t.	snipped chives	5 mL
dash	salt	dash
1	egg, well beaten	1

Melt margarine in a small skillet. Add hash-brown potatoes and chives. While stirring, cook over medium-low heat for 3 minutes. Sprinkle with salt. Pour in egg. Reduce heat to LOW. Lift potatoes slightly to allow egg to run under potatoes. Cover and cook until surface of egg is set but still shiny. Turn out onto serving plate.

Yield: 1 serving
Exchange, 1 serving: 1 medium-fat meat, 1 starch/bread
Calories, 1 serving: 166
Carbohydrates, 1 serving: 11

Tuna-Tip Stick-and-Dip Sandwiches

½ c.	tuna in water (drained and grated)	125 mL
¼ T.	low-calorie salad dressing	60 mL
1 T.	finely chopped dill pickle	15 mL
1 T.	finely chopped celery	15 mL
	salt and pepper to taste	
8	hard breadsticks	8

Combine tuna, salad dressing, dill pickle, celery, salt, and pepper in a bowl. Stir to mix. To eat: Dip the breadstick into mixture.

Yield: 8 servings
Exchange, 1 serving: ½ starch/bread, ½ lean meat
Calories, 1 serving: 64
Carbohydrates, 1 serving: 7

Wrangler Hamburgers

1 lb.	lean ground beef	500 g
1 c.	dry bread crumbs	250 mL
½ c.	finely chopped onion	125 mL
½ c.	tomato juice	125 mL
1	egg, slightly beaten	1
½ t.	salt	2 mL
¼ t.	black pepper	1 mL

Combine all ingredients in a bowl. With your hands or a spoon, work ingredients until thoroughly blended. Shape meat mixture into eight patties. Place patties on a broiler pan or hot grill. Broil 8 to 10 minutes. Then turn and brown other side.

Yield: 8 servings
Exchange, 1 serving: 1 medium-fat meat, ½ starch/bread
Calories, 1 serving: 159
Carbohydrates, 1 serving: 8

Round-up Hot Dogs

½ c.	shredded Cheddar cheese	125 mL
3 T.	sour pickle relish	45 mL
⅛ t.	black pepper	½ mL
8	hot dogs	8
8 slices	bacon	8 slices

Combine cheese, relish, and pepper in a bowl. Mix to blend. Slice hot dogs down the long side, not quite through. Stuff hot dogs with cheese mixture. Fry bacon slightly, but keep flexible, not crisp. Wrap each hot dog with a slice of bacon. Fasten each end of the bacon with a toothpick. Place hot dogs on a broiler or hot grill. Then broil for 3 to 4 minutes.

Yield: 8 servings
Exchange, 1 serving: 2½ high-fat meat
Calories, 1 serving: 240
Carbohydrates, 1 serving: negligible

Heifer Legs

1 lb.	ground beef	500 g
1	egg, well beaten	1
¼ c.	finely chopped onion	60 mL
1 t.	prepared yellow mustard	5 mL
½ t.	Worcestershire sauce	2 mL
	salt and pepper to taste	
½ c.	dry bread crumbs	125 mL
3 T.	vegetable oil	45 mL

Combine beef, egg, onion, mustard, Worcestershire sauce, salt, and pepper in a bowl. With your hands or a spoon, mix to blend. Divide meat into six equal portions. Shape each portion around wooden skewer or stick, leaving half of the stick showing as the thin leg. (Meat should look like the end of a lollipop.) Roll each leg in the bread crumbs, pressing slightly to coat each leg. Heat oil in a skillet. Then place legs in skillet and fry over medium heat. Turn to brown all sides. Continue cooking over low heat for 15 to 20 minutes or until done.

Yield: 6 servings
Exchange, 1 serving: 2 medium-fat meat, ⅓ starch/bread
Calories, 1 serving: 180
Carbohydrates, 1 serving: 5

Prairie Porcupines

1 lb.	ground beef	500 mL
½ c.	uncooked rice	125 mL
¼ c.	finely chopped onion	60 mL
1 t.	salt	5 mL
⅛ t.	black pepper	½ mL
10-oz. can	tomato soup	280-g can
½ c.	water	125 mL

Combine ground beef, uncooked rice, onion, salt, and pepper in a bowl. With your hands or a spoon, mix thoroughly. Shape meat mixture into eight balls. Place in casserole. Combine tomato soup and water in a bowl, stirring to mix. Then pour tomato sauce over meat balls. Cover and bake at 350 °F (175 °C) for an hour or until rice is tender.

Yield: 8 servings
Exchange, 1 serving: 1 medium-fat meat, ⅔ starch/bread
Calories, 1 serving: 165
Carbohydrates, 1 serving: 13

Farm Omelet

1	egg	1
1 T.	skim milk	15 mL
	salt and pepper to taste	
2 t.	low-calorie margarine	10 mL
¼ c.	shredded Cheddar cheese	60 mL

Combine egg, milk, salt, and pepper in a bowl. Beat until well blended but not foamy. Melt margarine in small skillet. Pour egg mixture into skillet and reduce heat. As the edges of the omelet start to thicken, lift edge of omelet and put a few drops of water under it. Cover and allow to cook over low heat. When egg is almost cooked but surface is still moist, add cheese. Loosen edges carefully, and fold in half. Return cover to pan and cook for a minute. Then slide omelet onto a warm plate.

Yield: 1 serving
Exchange, 1 serving: 2 high-fat meat
Calories, 1 serving: 194
Carbohydrates, 1 serving: negligible

Rustler's Beef

2 oz.	breakfast beef steak	58 g
½ t.	Worcestershire sauce	2 mL
⅛ t.	ground oregano	½ mL
½ t.	prepared yellow mustard	2 mL
¼	dill pickle	¼

Spray a small skillet with vegetable cooking oil. Heat slightly. Place beef steak in bottom of skillet. Brown slightly; then turn and brown the other side. Add Worcestershire sauce and oregano to skillet. Cover and cook for a minute. Remove beef steak to warmed plate. Spread with mustard. Then roll steak around dill pickle.

Yield: 1 serving
Exchange, 1 serving: 2 medium-fat meat
Calories, 1 serving: 135
Carbohydrates, 1 serving: negligible

Potato Pan Bread

1 env.	dry yeast	1 env.
¼ c.	warm water	60 mL
½ c.	instant mashed-potato flakes	125 mL
1¾ c.	warm water	440 mL
6 c.	all-purpose flour	1500 mL
2 T.	granulated sugar replacement	30 mL
2 t.	salt	10 mL
2 T.	low-calorie margarine, melted	30 mL

Sprinkle yeast over the ¼ c. (60 mL) of warm water. Stir and allow to soften for 5 minutes. Combine potato flakes and the 1¾ c. (440 mL) of warm water in a mixing bowl. Stir to blend. Cover and allow potato flakes to soften for 5 minutes. Combine yeast water and potato water. Reserve 2 T. (30 mL) of the flour. Stir sugar replacement, salt, and 3 c. (750 mL) of the flour into the yeast-potato mixture. With an electric beater, beat until smooth. Next, beat in melted margarine and remaining flour except the reserved 2 T. (30 mL). Then turn dough out onto a lighly floured surface. Knead quickly and lightly for about 5 minutes or until dough is smooth and elastic. Place dough in a greased bowl; then cover and allow to rise until doubled in size. Divide dough into two equal portions. Shape into round loaves. Place each loaf in a greased pie pan. Dust the tops of the loaves with the reserved flour. Cover and allow to rise again until doubled in size. Bake at 425 °F (220 °C) for 15 minutes; then reduce heat to 375 °F (190 °C) and finish baking for 30 more minutes or until done.

Yield: 2 loaves or 30 servings
Exchange, 1 serving: 1 starch/bread
Calories, 1 serving: 82
Carbohydrates, 1 serving: 16

Hot Cross Buns

1 env.	dry yeast	1 env.
1 T.	sugar replacement	15 mL
1 c.	skim milk, lukewarm	250 mL
3¾ c.	all-purpose flour	940 mL
¼ c.	currants	60 mL
¼ c.	low-calorie margarine	60 mL
⅓ c.	granulated sugar replacement	90 mL
¼ t.	salt	1 mL
1	egg, well beaten	1

Dissolve yeast and sugar replacement in lukewarm skim milk. Add half of the flour. Beat until smooth and elastic. Cover and allow to rise for an hour. Combine currants and remaining flour in a bowl. Toss to coat currants. Cream margarine and granulated sugar replacement together; then add salt. Stir into flour-yeast dough. Add egg and currants-flour mixture. Stir to mix. Then turn out onto a lightly floured surface. Knead lightly. Place in a greased bowl. Cover and allow to rise for about 2 hours or until doubled in size. Shape into 24 round buns; then place in well-greased shallow pans. Cover and allow to rise again for about an hour or until light. Brush tops with water. With a sharp knife, cut a cross on the top of each bun. Bake at 425 °F (220 °C) for 20 minutes or until done.

Yield: 24 servings
Exchange, 1 serving: 1 starch/bread
Calories, 1 serving: 76
Carbohydrates, 1 serving: 14

Snow Biscuits

1 env.	dry yeast	1 env.
¾ c.	warm water	190 mL
2 c.	all-purpose flour	500 mL
1 T.	granulated sugar replacement	15 mL
½ t.	salt	2 mL
1 T.	low-calorie margarine, melted	15 mL

Sprinkle yeast over bowl of warm water. Stir and then allow to soften for 5 minutes. Combine flour, sugar replacement, and salt in a mixing bowl. Add softened yeast and melted margarine. Stir to mix. (Dough will be soft.) Turn out dough onto lightly floured surface. Knead dough quickly and lightly for about 10 minutes or until smooth and elastic. Roll out until ½ in. (1.25 cm) thick. Cut with a 2-in. (5-cm) floured biscuit cutter. Place biscuits in a greased pan. Cover and allow to rise until doubled in size. Prick tops with a fork. Then bake at 425 °F (220 °C) for 20 minutes or until done.

Yield: 16 biscuits
Exchange, 1 serving: 1 starch/bread
Calories, 1 serving: 72
Carbohydrates, 1 serving: 13

English Crumpets

2 env.	dry yeast	2 env.
1 qt.	warm water	1 L
4 c.	all-purpose flour	1000 mL
1 T.	salt	15 mL

Sprinkle yeast over bowl of warm water. Stir and then allow yeast to soften for 5 minutes. Add flour and salt. Beat well. Cover and allow to rise until doubled in size. Beat well again. Half-fill greased muffin or egg rings, placed on a slightly greased griddle heated to a medium temperature. When the bubbles of the batter rise to the top and break, making holes through the crumpets from top to bottom, reduce to a low heat and fry until crumpets are dry on top and begin to shrink at the edges.

Yield: 12 crumpets
Exchange, 1 crumpet: 2 starch/bread
Calories, 1 crumpet: 140
Carbohydrates, 1 crumpet: 29

Angel Pudding

4	eggs	4
¼ c.	granulated sugar replacement	60 mL
¼ t.	salt	1 mL
3 c.	skim milk	750 mL
1 t.	vanilla extract	5 mL
6 (½ in.) slices	angel food cake	6 (1.25 cm) slices
10 T.	prepared nondairy whipped topping	150 mL

Preheat oven to 350 °F (175 °C). Grease the bottom of a 10 × 6 in. (25 × 16 cm) baking pan. Beat eggs slightly; then add sugar replacement and salt, and beat well. Gradually beat in milk and vanilla. Pour just enough of this pudding mixture into the bottom of the prepared pan to cover. Lay cake slices on top of pudding in a single layer, covering the bottom of the pan. Pour remaining pudding over cake. Bake for 45 minutes or until knife inserted in center comes out clean. Cool to room temperature. Chill and then cut into 10 pieces to serve. Top each piece with 1 T. (15 mL) of whipped topping.

Yield: 10 servings
Exchange, 1 serving: ½ medium-fat meat, ⅓ skim milk
Calories, 1 serving: 107
Carbohydrates, 1 serving: 4

Raisin Tarts

8	individual frozen unbaked tart shells	8
1½ c.	raisins	375 mL
2 T.	chopped pecans	30 mL
1 T.	lemon juice	15 mL

Line tart pans as described on tart-shell package. Cover raisins with water; then bring to a boil. Allow to completely cool. Drain thoroughly. Combine drained raisins, pecans, and lemon juice in bowl. Mix. Fill tart shells. Bake at 400 °F (200 °C) for 15 to 20 minutes.

Yield: 8 servings
Exchange, 1 serving: 1 starch/bread, 1⅓ fruit, 1 fat
Calories, 1 serving: 203
Carbohydrates, 1 serving: 33

EXCHANGE LISTS

FOR MEAL PLANNING

The reason for dividing food into six different groups is that foods vary in their carbohydrate, protein, fat, and calorie content. Each exchange list contains foods that are alike – each choice contains about the same amount of carbohydrate, protein, fat, and calories.

The following chart shows the amount of these nutrients in one serving from each exchange list.

Exchange List	Carbohydrate (grams)	Protein (grams)	Fat (grams)	Calories
Starch/Bread	15	3	trace	80
Meat				
Lean	--	7	3	55
Medium-Fat	–	7	5	75
High-Fat	–	7	8	100
Vegetable	5	2	–	25
Fruit	15	–	–	60
Milk				
Skim	12	8	trace	90
Low-fat	12	8	5	120
Whole	12	8	8	150
Fat	–	–	5	45

As you read the exchange lists, you will notice that one choice often is a larger amount of food than another choice from the same list. Because foods are so different, each food is measured or weighed so the amount of carbohydrate, protein, fat, and calories is the same in each choice.

You will notice symbols on some foods in the exchange groups. Foods that are high in fiber (3 grams or more per normal serving) have this symbol. High fiber foods are good for you. It is important to eat more of these foods.

Foods that are high in sodium (400 milligrams or more of sodium per normal serving) have this symbol. It's a good idea to limit your intake of high salt foods, especially if you have high blood pressure.

If you have a favorite food that is not included in any of these groups, ask your dietitian about it. That food can probably be worked into your meal plan, at least now and then.

*The exchange lists are the basis of a meal planning system designed by a committee of the American Diabetes Association and the American Dietetic Association. While designed primarily for people with diabetes and others who must follow special diets, the exchange lists are based on principles of good nutrition that apply to everyone. ©1986 American Diabetes Association, American Dietetic Association.

1
Starch/Bread List

ach item in this list contains approximately 15 grams of carbohydrate, 3 grams of protein, a trace of fat, and 80 calories. Whole grain products average about 2 grams of fiber per serving. Some foods are higher in fiber. Those foods that contain 3 or more grams of fiber per serving are identified with the fiber symbol ✍

You can choose your starch exchanges from any of the items on this list. If you want to eat a starch food that is not on this list, the general rule is that:

- 1/2 cup of cereal, grain or pasta is one serving
- 1 ounce of a bread product is one serving

Your dietitian can help you be more exact.

CEREALS/GRAINS/PASTA

✍ Bran cereals, concentrated	1/3 cup
✍ Bran cereals, flaked (such as Bran Buds,® All Bran®)	1/2 cup
Bulgur (cooked)	1/2 cup
Cooked cereals	1/2 cup
Cornmeal (dry)	2 1/2 Tbsp.
Grapenuts	3 Tbsp.
Grits (cooked)	1/2 cup
Other ready-to-eat unsweetened cereals	3/4 cup
Pasta (cooked)	1/2 cup
Puffed cereal	1 1/2 cup
Rice, white or brown (cooked)	1/3 cup
Shredded wheat	1/2 cup
✍ Wheat germ	3 Tbsp.

DRIED BEANS/PEAS/LENTILS

✍ Beans and peas (cooked) (such as kidney, white, split, blackeye)	1/3 cup
✍ Lentils (cooked)	1/3 cup
✍ Baked beans	1/4 cup

STARCHY VEGETABLES

✍ Corn	1/2 cup
✍ Corn on cob, 6 in. long	1
✍ Lima beans	1/2 cup
✍ Peas, green (canned or frozen)	1/2 cup
✍ Plantain	1/2 cup
Potato, baked	1 small (3 oz.)
Potato, mashed	1/2 cup
Squash, winter (acorn, butternut)	3/4 cup
Yam, sweet potato, plain	1/3 cup

BREAD

Bagel	1/2 (1 oz.)
Bread sticks, crisp, 4 in. long x 1/2 in.	2 (2/3 oz.)
Croutons, low fat	1 cup
English muffin	1/2
Frankfurter or hamburger bun	1/2 (1 oz.)
Pita, 6 in. across	1/2
Plain roll, small	1 (1 oz.)
Raisin, unfrosted	1 slice (1 oz.)
✍ Rye, pumpernickel	1 slice (1 oz.)
Tortilla, 6 in. across	1
White (including French, Italian)	1 slice (1 oz.)
Whole wheat	1 slice (1 oz.)

CRACKERS/SNACKS

Animal crackers	8
Graham crackers, 2 1/2 in. square	3
Matzoth	3/4 oz.
Melba toast	5 slices
Oyster crackers	24
Popcorn (popped, no fat added)	3 cups
Pretzels	3/4 oz.
Rye crisp, 2 in. x 3 1/2 in.	4
Saltine-type crackers	6
Whole wheat crackers, no fat added (crisp breads, such as Finn®, Kavli®, Wasa®)	2-4 slices (3/4 oz.)

STARCH FOODS PREPARED WITH FAT

(Count as 1 starch/bread serving, plus 1 fat serving.)

Biscuit, 2 1/2 in. across	1
Chow mein noodles	1/2 cup
Corn bread, 2 in. cube	1 (2 oz.)
Cracker, round butter type	6
French fried potatoes, 2 in. to 3 1/2 in. long	10 (1 1/2 oz.)
Muffin, plain, small	1
Pancake, 4 in. across	2
Stuffing, bread (prepared)	1/4 cup
Taco shell, 6 in. across	2
Waffle, 4 1/2 in. square	1
Whole wheat crackers, fat added (such as Triscuits®)	4-6 (1 oz.)

✍ *3 grams or more of fiber per serving*

2
Meat List

Each serving of meat and substitutes on this list contains about 7 grams of protein. The amount of fat and number of calories varies, depending on what kind of meat or substitute you choose. The list is divided into three parts based on the amount of fat and calories: lean meat, medium-fat meat, and high-fat meat. One ounce (one meat exchange) of each of these includes:

	Carbohydrate (grams)	Protein (grams)	Fat (grams)	Calories
Lean	0	7	3	55
Medium-Fat	0	7	5	75
High-Fat	0	7	8	100

You are encouraged to use more lean and medium-fat meat, poultry, and fish in your meal plan. This will help decrease your fat intake, which may help decrease your risk for heart disease. The items from the high-fat group are high in saturated fat, cholesterol, and calories. You should limit your choices from the high-fat group to three (3) times per week. Meat and substitutes do not contribute any fiber to your meal plan.

TIPS

1. Bake, roast, broil, grill, or boil these foods rather than frying them with added fat.

2. Use a nonstick pan spray or a nonstick pan to brown or fry these foods.

3. Trim off visible fat before and after cooking.

4. Do not add flour, bread crumbs, coating mixes, or fat to these foods when preparing them.

5. Weigh meat after removing bones and fat, and after cooking. Three ounces of cooked meat is about equal to 4 ounces of raw meat. Some examples of meat portions are:

2 ounces meat (2 meat exchanges) =
1 small chicken leg or thigh
½ cup cottage cheese or tuna

3 ounces meat (3 meat exchanges) =
1 medium pork chop
1 small hamburger
½ of a whole chicken breast
1 unbreaded fish fillet
cooked meat about the size of a deck of cards

6. Restaurants usually serve prime cuts of meat, which are high in fat and calories.

🐟 Meats and meat substitutes that have 400 milligrams or more of sodium per exchange are indicated with this symbol.

LEAN MEAT AND SUBSTITUTES
(One exchange is equal to any one of the following items.)

Beef: USDA Good or Choice grades of lean beef, such as round, sirloin, and flank steak; tenderloin; and chipped beef 🐟 1 oz.

Pork: Lean pork, such as fresh ham; canned, cured or boiled ham 🐟; Canadian bacon 🐟, tenderloin. 1 oz.

Veal: All cuts are lean except for veal cutlets (ground or cubed). Examples of lean veal are chops and roasts. 1 oz.

Poultry: Chicken, turkey, Cornish hen (without skin) 1 oz.

Fish:
All fresh and frozen fish 1 oz.
Crab, lobster, scallops, shrimp, clams (fresh or canned in water 🐟) 2 oz.
Oysters 6 medium
Tuna 🐟 (canned in water) 1/4 cup
Herring (uncreamed or smoked) 1 oz.
Sardines (canned) 2 medium

Wild Game:
Venison, rabbit, squirrel 1 oz.
Pheasant, duck, goose (without skin) 1 oz.

Cheese:	Any cottage cheese	1/4 cup
	Grated parmesan	2 Tbsp.
	Diet cheeses 🔳 (with less than 55 calories per ounce)	1 oz.
Other:	95% fat-free luncheon meat	1 oz.
	Egg whites	3 whites
	Egg substitutes with less than 55 calories per 1/4 cup	1/4 cup

MEDIUM-FAT MEAT AND SUBSTITUTES
(One exchange is equal to any one of the following items.)

Beef:	Most beef products fall into this category. Examples are: all ground beef, roast (rib, chuck, rump), steak (cubed, Porterhouse, T-bone), and meatloaf.	1 oz.
Pork:	Most pork products fall into this category. Examples are: chops, loin roast, Boston butt, cutlets.	1 oz.
Lamb:	Most lamb products fall into this category. Examples are: chops, leg, and roast.	1 oz.
Veal:	Cutlet (ground or cubed, unbreaded)	1 oz.
Poultry:	Chicken (with skin), domestic duck or goose (well-drained of fat), ground turkey	1 oz.
Fish:	Tuna 🔳 (canned in oil and drained)	1/4 cup
	Salmon 🔳 (canned)	1/4 cup
Cheese:	Skim or part-skim milk cheeses, such as:	
	Ricotta	1/4 cup
	Mozzarella	1 oz.
	Diet cheeses 🔳 (with 56-80 calories per ounce)	1 oz.
Other:	86% fat-free luncheon meat 🔳	1 oz.
	Egg (high in cholesterol, limit to 3 per week)	1
	Egg substitutes with 56-80 calories per 1/4 cup	1/4 cup
	Tofu (2 1/2 in. x 2 3/4 in. x 1 in.)	4 oz.
	Liver, heart, kidney, sweetbreads (high in cholesterol)	1 oz.

HIGH-FAT MEAT AND SUBSTITUTES
Remember, these items are high in saturated fat, cholesterol, and calories, and should be used only three (3) times per week.
(One exchange is equal to any one of the following items.)

Beef:	Most USDA Prime cuts of beef, such as ribs, corned beef 🔳	1 oz.
Pork:	Spareribs, ground pork, pork sausage 🔳 (patty or link)	1 oz.
Lamb:	Patties (ground lamb)	1 oz.
Fish:	Any fried fish product	1 oz.
Cheese:	All regular cheeses 🔳 , such as American, Blue, Cheddar, Monterey, Swiss	1 oz.
Other:	Luncheon meat 🔳 , such as bologna, salami, pimento loaf	1 oz.
	Sausage 🔳 , such as Polish, Italian	1 oz.
	Knockwurst, smoked	1 oz.
	Bratwurst 🔳	1 oz.
	Frankfurter 🔳 (turkey or chicken)	1 frank (10/lb.)
	Peanut butter (contains unsaturated fat)	1 Tbsp.

Count as one high-fat meat plus one fat exchange:

| Frankfurter 🔳 (beef, pork, or combination) | 1 frank (10/lb.) |

🔳 *400 mg or more of sodium per exchange*

3
Vegetable List 🌾

Each vegetable serving on this list contains about 5 grams of carbohydrate, 2 grams of protein, and 25 calories. Vegetables contain 2-3 grams of dietary fiber. Vegetables which contain 400 mg of sodium per serving are identified with a 🔫 symbol.

Vegetables are a good source of vitamins and minerals. Fresh and frozen vegetables have more vitamins and less added salt. Rinsing canned vegetables will remove much of the salt.

Unless otherwise noted, the serving size for vegetables (one vegetable exchange) is:

1/2 cup of cooked vegetables or vegetable juice
1 cup of raw vegetables

Artichoke (1/2 medium)
Asparagus
Beans (green, wax, Italian)
Bean sprouts
Beets
Broccoli
Brussels sprouts
Cabbage, cooked
Carrots

Cauliflower
Eggplant
Greens (collard, mustard, turnip)
Kohlrabi
Leeks
Mushrooms, cooked
Okra
Onions
Pea pods
Peppers (green)

Rutabaga
Sauerkraut 🔫
Spinach, cooked
Summer squash (crookneck)
Tomato (one large)

Tomato/vegetable juice 🔫
Turnips
Water chestnuts
Zucchini, cooked

Starchy vegetables such as corn, peas, and potatoes are found on the Starch/Bread List.

4
Fruit List

Each item on this list contains about 15 grams of carbohydrate, and 60 calories. Fresh, frozen, and dry fruits have about 2 grams of fiber per serving. Fruits that have 3 or more grams of fiber per serving have a 🍃 symbol. Fruit juices contain very little dietary fiber.

The carbohydrate and calorie content for a fruit serving are based on the usual serving of the most commonly eaten fruits. Use fresh fruits or fruits frozen or canned without sugar added. Whole fruit is more filling than fruit juice and may be a better choice for those who are trying to lose weight. Unless otherwise noted, the serving size for one fruit serving is:

1/2 cup of fresh fruit or fruit juice
1/4 cup of dried fruit

FRESH, FROZEN, AND UNSWEETENED CANNED FRUIT

Apple (raw, 2 in. across)	1 apple
Applesauce (unsweetened)	1/2 cup
Apricots (medium, raw) or	4 apricots
Apricots (canned)	1/2 cup, or 4 halves
Banana (9 in. long)	1/2 banana
🍃 Blackberries (raw)	3/4 cup
🍃 Blueberries (raw)	3/4 cup
Cantaloupe (5 in. across) (cubes)	1/3 melon 1 cup
Cherries (large, raw)	12 cherries
Cherries (canned)	1/2 cup
Figs (raw, 2 in. across)	2 figs
Fruit cocktail (canned)	1/2 cup
Grapefruit (medium)	1/2 grapefruit
Grapefruit (segments)	3/4 cup
Grapes (small)	15 grapes
Honeydew melon (medium) (cubes)	1/8 melon 1 cup
Kiwi (large)	1 kiwi
Mandarin oranges	3/4 cup
Mango (small)	1/2 mango
🍃 Nectarine (1 1/2 in. across)	1 nectarine
Orange (2 1/2 in. across)	1 orange
Papaya	1 cup
Peach (2 3/4 in. across)	1 peach, or 3/4 cup
Peaches (canned)	1/2 cup, or 2 halves
Pear	1/2 large, or 1 small
Pears (canned)	1/2 cup or 2 halves
Persimmon (medium, native)	2 persimmons
Pineapple (raw)	3/4 cup

🔫 400 mg or more of sodium per exchange   🍃 3 or more grams of fiber per serving

Pineapple (canned)	1/3 cup	
Plum (raw, 2 in. across)	2 plums	
☞ Pomegranate	1/2 pomegranate	
☞ Raspberries (raw)	1 cup	
☞ Strawberries (raw, whole)	1 1/4 cup	
Tangerine (2 1/2 in. across)	2 tangerines	
Watermelon (cubes)	1 1/4 cup	

DRIED FRUIT

☞ Apples	4 rings
☞ Apricots	7 halves
Dates	2 1/2 medium
☞ Figs	1 1/2
☞ Prunes	3 medium
Raisins	2 Tbsp.

FRUIT JUICE

Apple juice/cider	1/2 cup
Cranberry juice cocktail	1/3 cup
Grapefruit juice	1/2 cup
Grape juice	1/3 cup
Orange juice	1/2 cup
Pineapple juice	1/2 cup
Prune juice	1/3 cup

5
Milk List

Each serving of milk or milk products on this list contains about 12 grams of carbohydrate and 8 grams of protein. The amount of fat in milk is measured in percent (%) of butterfat. The calories vary, depending on what kind of milk you choose. The list is divided into three parts based on the amount of fat and calories: skim/very lowfat milk, lowfat milk, and whole milk. One serving (one milk exchange) of each of these includes:

	Carbohydrate (grams)	Protein (grams)	Fat (grams)	Calories
Skim/Very Lowfat	12	8	trace	90
Lowfat	12	8	5	120
Whole	12	8	8	150

Milk is the body's main source of calcium, the mineral needed for growth and repair of bones. Yogurt is also a good source of calcium. Yogurt and many dry or powdered milk products have different amounts of fat. If you have questions about a particular item, read the label to find out the fat and calorie content.

Milk is good to drink, but it can also be added to cereal, and to other foods. Many tasty dishes such as sugar-free pudding are made with milk.

SKIM AND VERY LOWFAT MILK

skim milk	1 cup
1/2% milk	1 cup
1% milk	1 cup
lowfat buttermilk	1 cup
evaporated skim milk	1/2 cup
dry nonfat milk	1/3 cup
plain nonfat yogurt	8 oz.

LOWFAT MILK

2% milk	1 cup fluid
plain lowfat yogurt (with added nonfat milk solids)	8 oz.

WHOLE MILK

The whole milk group has much more fat per serving than the skim and lowfat groups. Whole milk has more than 3 1/4% butterfat. Try to limit your choices from the whole milk group as much as possible.

whole milk	1 cup
evaporated whole milk	1/2 cup
whole plain yogurt	8 oz.

☞ 3 or more grams of fiber per serving

6
Fat List

Each serving on the fat list contains about 5 grams of fat and 45 calories.

The foods on the fat list contain mostly fat, although some items may also contain a small amount of protein. All fats are high in calories and should be carefully measured. Everyone should modify fat intake by eating unsaturated fats instead of saturated fats. The sodium content of these foods varies widely. Check the label for sodium information.

UNSATURATED FATS

Avocado	1/8 medium
Margarine	1 tsp.
* Margarine, diet	1 Tbsp.
Mayonnaise	1 tsp.
* Mayonnaise, reduced-calorie	1 Tbsp.

Nuts and Seeds:

Almonds, dry roasted	6 whole
Cashews, dry roasted	1 Tbsp.
Pecans	2 whole
Peanuts	20 small or 10 large
Walnuts	2 whole
Other nuts	1 Tbsp.
Seeds, pine nuts, sun-flower (without shells)	1 Tbsp.
Pumpkin seeds	2 tsp.

Oil (corn, cottonseed, safflower, soybean, sunflower, olive, peanut)	1 tsp.
* Olives	10 small or 5 large
Salad dressing, mayonnaise-type	2 tsp.
Salad dressing, mayonnaise-type, reduced-calorie	1 Tbsp.
* Salad dressing (all varieties)	1 Tbsp.

🧂 Salad dressing, reduced-calorie	2 Tbsp.

(Two tablespoons of low-calorie salad dressing is a free food.)

SATURATED FATS

Butter	1 tsp.
* Bacon	1 slice
Chitterlings	1/2 ounce
Coconut, shredded	2 Tbsp.
Coffee whitener, liquid	2 Tbsp.
Coffee whitener, powder	4 tsp.
Cream (light, coffee, table)	2 Tbsp.
Cream, sour	2 Tbsp.
Cream (heavy, whipping)	1 Tbsp.
Cream cheese	1 Tbsp.
* Salt pork	1/4 ounce

---

* *If more than one or two servings are eaten, these foods have 400 mg. or more of sodium.*

🧂 *400 mg. or more of sodium per serving.*

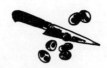

Snack Product Information

Food manufacturers now include nutritional information on the labels of their products. This information can be very useful to anyone using the American Diabetes Association's exchange lists or the calorie/carbohydrate method in their diets. The labels show the number of calories and the grams of protein, carbohydrates, and fat in each serving. Most of the labels resemble the example that follows.

NUTRITIONAL INFORMATION PER SERVING
Servings per container: 12
Serving size (Cookie): 3
Calories per serving: 170
Protein: 2 g
Carbohydrates: 22 g
Fat: 7 g

With this information you can work out the food exchange on any product. The following exchange list is needed for calculations.

Exchange	Calories	Carbohydrate (grams)	Protein (grams)	Fat (grams)
Milk				
Whole	150	12	8	8
2%	120	12	8	5
Skim	90	12	8	0
Vegetable	25	5	2	0
Fruit	60	15	0	0
Starch/Bread	80	15	3	0
Meat				
Lean	55	0	7	3
Medium-fat	75	0	7	5
High-fat	100	0	7	8
Fat	45	0	0	5

Compare the nutrient value on the label with the nutrient values on the exchange list. Count whole and nearest half exchanges.

	Exchange	C	P	F
1. List the grams of carbohydrates, proteins, and fat per serving.		22	2	7
2. Subtract carbohydrates first. Bread exchange has 15 carbohydrates + 3 protein.	1 bread	−15	−3	
		7	0	7
3. Compare the next nearest carbohydrate exchange. Fruit has 15.	½ fruit	−7		
		0	0	7
4. Compare the fat exchange.	1 fat			−5
				2

You have 2 grams of fat left, or approximately ½ fat exchange; therefore, your exchange on one serving of this product is equivalent to 1 starch/bread, ½ fruit, and 1½ fat.

5. Check with calories

1 starch/bread = 80 calories
½ fruit = 30 calories
1½ fat = 67 calories

Total: 177 calories (Product information states 170)

It's important to realize that most exchanges figured on foods will vary because the averages are taken for calculating the original exchange value.

Convenience Product Lists

The retail convenience product lists that follow are reprinted with permission of Campbell Soup Company; Carnation Company; The Dannon Company, Inc.; The Estee Corporation; Health Valley Foods; Hodgson Mill Enterprises, Inc.; Pepperidge Farm; and The Pillsbury Company.

Remember these are only general reference lists. Many of the products' ingredients vary from area to area, and from season to season. You *must* check the products' labels for the most recently updated information on serving size, calories, carbohydrates, protein, and fat.

Campbell Soup Products

CAMPBELL'S CONDENSED SOUPS

Beef
Serving Size: 8 oz. (prepared)
Calories, 1 serving: 80
Exchange, 1 serving: 1 vegetable
½ bread
½ lean meat

Beef Noodle
Serving Size: 8 oz. (prepared)
Calories, 1 serving: 70
Exchange, 1 serving: ½ bread
½ lean meat
½ fat

Beef Noodle, Homestyle
Serving Size: 8 oz. (prepared)
Calories, 1 serving: 80
Exchange, 1 serving: ½ bread
1 lean meat

Chicken Alphabet
Serving Size: 8 oz. (prepared)
Calories, 1 serving: 80
Exchange, 1 serving: ½ bread
½ lean meat
½ fat

Chicken, Cream of
Serving Size: 8 oz. (prepared)
Calories, 1 serving: 110
Exchange, 1 serving: ½ bread
½ lean meat
1 fat

Chicken Noodle
Serving Size: 8 oz. (prepared)
Calories, 1 serving: 70
Exchange, 1 serving: ½ bread
½ fat

Chicken Noodle, Homestyle
Serving Size: 8 oz. (prepared)
Calories, 1 serving: 70
Exchange, 1 serving: ½ bread
½ fat

Chicken with Rice
Serving Size: 8 oz. (prepared)
Calories, 1 serving: 60
Exchange, 1 serving: ½ bread
½ fat

Clam Chowder (Manhattan Style)
Serving Size: 8 oz. (prepared)
Calories, 1 serving: 70
Exchange, 1 serving: 1 vegetable
½ bread
½ fat

**Clam Chowder, New England
(Made with Milk—Whole)**
Serving Size: 8 oz. (prepared)
Calories, 1 serving: 150
Exchange, 1 serving: ½ milk
½ bread
½ lean meat

Minestrone
Serving Size: 8 oz. (prepared)
Calories, 1 serving: 80
Exchange, 1 serving: 1 vegetable
½ bread
½ fat

**Oyster Stew (Made with
Milk—Whole)**
Serving Size: 8 oz. (prepared)
Calories, 1 serving: 150
Exchange, 1 serving: ½ milk
½ bread
½ lean meat
½ fat

**Potato, Cream of (Made with Water &
Milk—Whole)**
Serving Size: 8 oz. (prepared)
Calories, 1 serving: 110
Exchange, 1 serving: ¼ milk
½ bread
½ fat

Split Peas with Ham & Bacon
Serving Size: 8 oz. (prepared)
Calories, 1 serving: 160
Exchange, 1 serving: 1½ bread
½ lean meat
½ fat

Tomato
Serving Size: 8 oz. (prepared)
Calories, 1 serving: 90
Exchange, 1 serving: 1 bread
½ fat

Tomato (Made with Milk—Whole)
Serving Size: 8 oz. (prepared)
Calories, 1 serving: 160
Exchange, 1 serving: ½ milk
1 bread
½ fat

Tomato Rice, Old Fashioned
Serving Size: 8 oz. (prepared)
Calories, 1 serving: 110
Exchange, 1 serving: 1½ bread
½ fat

Turkey Noodle
Serving Size: 8 oz. (prepared)
Calories, 1 serving: 60
Exchange, 1 serving: ½ bread
½ fat

Turkey Vegetable
Serving Size: 8 oz. (prepared)
Calories, 1 serving: 70
Exchange, 1 serving: 1 vegetable
　　　　　　　　　½ bread
　　　　　　　　　½ fat

Vegetable, Old Fashioned
Serving Size: 8 oz. (prepared)
Calories, 1 serving: 60
Exchange, 1 serving: 1 vegetable
　　　　　　　　　½ bread
　　　　　　　　　½ fat

Vegetable
Serving Size: 8 oz. (prepared)
Calories, 1 serving: 80
Exchange, 1 serving: 1 vegetable
　　　　　　　　　½ bread
　　　　　　　　　½ fat

Vegetable, Beef
Serving Size: 8 oz. (prepared)
Calories, 1 serving: 70
Exchange, 1 serving: 1 vegetable
　　　　　　　　　½ lean meat
　　　　　　　　　½ fat

CREAMY NATURAL CONDENSED SOUPS (MADE WITH MILK—WHOLE)

Broccoli
Serving Size: 8 oz. (prepared)
Calories, 1 serving: 140
Exchange, 1 serving: ½ milk
　　　　　　　　　1 vegetable
　　　　　　　　　½ fat

Potato
Serving Size: 8 oz. (prepared)
Calories, 1 serving: 220
Exchange, 1 serving: ½ milk
　　　　　　　　　1 vegetable
　　　　　　　　　½ bread
　　　　　　　　　2 fat

Cauliflower
Serving Size: 8 oz. (prepared)
Calories, 1 serving: 200
Exchange, 1 serving: ½ milk
　　　　　　　　　1 vegetable
　　　　　　　　　½ bread
　　　　　　　　　1½ fat

Tomato
Serving Size: 8 oz. (prepared)
Calories, 1 serving: 190
Exchange, 1 serving: ½ milk
　　　　　　　　　1½ vegetable
　　　　　　　　　½ bread
　　　　　　　　　1 fat

CAMPBELL'S SOUP FOR ONE

Old Fashioned Bean with Ham
Serving Size: 11 oz. (prepared)
Calories, 1 serving: 220
Exchange, 1 serving: 2 bread
　　　　　　　　　½ lean meat
　　　　　　　　　1 fat

Barly Vegetable Beef & Bacon
Serving Size: 11 oz. (prepared)
Calories, 1 serving: 160
Exchange, 1 serving: 1 vegetable
　　　　　　　　　1 bread
　　　　　　　　　½ lean meat
　　　　　　　　　1 fat

CAMPBELL'S CHUNKY SOUPS (INDIVIDUAL SERVICE SIZE)

Chunky Beef
Serving Size: 10¾ (undiluted ounces)
Calories, 1 serving: 190
Exchange, 1 serving: 1½ bread
　　　　　　　　　1½ lean meat

Chunky Stroganoff
Serving Size: 10¾ (undiluted ounces)
Calories, 1 serving: 300
Exchange, 1 serving: 2 bread
　　　　　　　　　1½ lean meat
　　　　　　　　　2 fat

Chunky Old Fashioned Vegetable Beef
Serving Size: 10¾ (undiluted ounces)
Calories, 1 serving: 180
Exchange, 1 serving: 1 vegetable
 1 bread
 1 lean meat
 ½ fat

Chunky Steak 'n Potato
Serving Size: 10¾ (undiluted ounces)
Calories, 1 serving: 200
Exchange, 1 serving: 1½ bread
 1½ lean meat

Chunky Vegetable
Serving Size: 10¾ (undiluted ounces)
Calories, 1 serving: 140
Exchange, 1 serving: 1 milk
 1 bread
 1 fat

Chunky Fisherman Chowder
Serving Size: 10¾ (undiluted ounces)
Calories, 1 serving: 260
Exchange, 1 serving: 1½ bread
 1½ lean meat
 2 fat

Chunky Old Fashioned Chicken
Serving Size: 10¾ (undiluted ounces)
Calories, 1 serving: 170
Exchange, 1 serving: 1½ bread
 1 lean meat
 ½ fat

CAMPBELL'S CHUNKY SOUPS (19-OUNCE SIZE)

Chunky Beef
Serving Size: ½ can (undiluted
 ounces—9½)
Calories, 1 serving: 170
Exchange, 1 serving: 1 vegetable
 1 bread
 1½ lean meat
 ½ fat

Chunky Chili Beef
Serving Size: ½ can (undiluted
 ounces—9¾)
Calories, 1 serving: 260
Exchange, 1 serving: 2 bread
 2 lean meat

Chunky Old Fashioned Bean with Ham
Serving Size: ½ can (undiluted
 ounces—9⅝)
Calories, 1 serving: 260
Exchange, 1 serving: 2 bread
 1½ lean meat
 1 fat

CAMPBELL'S BEANS

Barbecue Beans
Serving Size: 7⅞ ounces
Calories, 1 serving: 250
Exchange, 1 serving: 3 bread
 1 fat

Beans & Franks in Tomato & Molasses Sauce
Serving Size: 7⅞ ounces
Calories, 1 serving: 360
Exchange, 1 serving: 3 bread
 1 lean meat
 2 fat

Home Style Beans
Serving Size: 8 ounces
Calories, 1 serving: 270
Exchange, 1 serving: 3½ bread
1 fat

Pork & Beans in Tomato Sauce
Serving Size: 8 ounces
Calories, 1 serving: 240
Exchange, 1 serving: 3 bread
1 fat

Old Fashioned Beans in Brown Sugar and Molasses Sauce
Serving Size: 8 ounces
Calories, 1 serving: 270
Exchange, 1 serving: 3½ bread
1 fat

CAMPBELL'S JUICES

Tomato Juice
Serving Size: 6 ounces
Calories, 1 serving: 35
Exchange, 1 serving: 1 fruit

"V-8" Vegetable Juice, No-Salt-Added
Serving Size: 6 ounces
Calories, 1 serving: 40
Exchange, 1 serving: 1 fruit

"V-8" Vegetable Juice
Serving Size: 6 ounces
Calories, 1 serving: 35
Exchange, 1 serving: 1 fruit

"V-8" Spicy Hot Vegetable Juice
Serving Size: 6 ounces
Calories, 1 serving: 35
Exchange, 1 serving: 1 fruit

FRANCO-AMERICAN PRODUCTS

Beef Ravioli in Meat Sauce
Serving Size: 7½ ounces
Calories, 1 serving: 230
Exchange, 1 serving: 1 vegetable
2 bread
½ lean meat
½ fat

Macaroni & Cheese
Serving Size: 7⅜ ounces
Calories, 1 serving: 170
Exchange, 1 serving: 1½ bread
½ lean meat
1 fat

Beef Raviolios in Meat Sauce
Serving Size: 7½ ounces
Calories, 1 serving: 250
Exchange, 1 serving: 1 vegetable
2 bread
½ lean meat
1 fat

Spaghetti in Meat Sauce
Serving Size: 7½ ounces
Calories, 1 serving: 210
Exchange, 1 serving: 1 vegetable
1½ bread
½ lean meat
1 fat

Elbo Macaroni & Cheese
Serving Size: 7⅜ ounces
Calories, 1 serving: 170
Exchange, 1 serving: 1½ bread
½ lean meat
1 fat

Spaghettios in Tomato and Cheese Sauce
Serving Size: 7⅜ ounces
Calories, 1 serving: 170
Exchange, 1 serving: 1 vegetable
2 bread
½ fat

Au Jus Gravy
Serving Size: 2 ounces
Calories, 1 serving: 25
Exchange, 1 serving: ½ fat

Beef Gravy
Serving Size: 2 ounces
Calories, 1 serving: 25
Exchange, 1 serving: ½ fat

Chicken Gravy
Serving Size: 2 ounces
Calories, 1 serving: 50
Exchange, 1 serving: 1 fat

Pork Gravy
Serving Size: 2 ounces
Calories, 1 serving: 40
Exchange, 1 serving: 1 fat

SWANSON CANNED PRODUCTS

Chunk White and Dark Chicken, in Water
Serving Size: 2½ ounces
Calories, 1 serving: 100
Exchange, 1 serving: 2 lean meat

Chunk Premium White Chicken
Serving Size: 2½ ounces
Calories, 1 serving: 90
Exchange, 1 serving: 2 lean meat

Chunk Style Mixin' Chicken
Serving Size: 2½ ounces
Calories, 1 serving: 130
Exchange, 1 serving: 2 lean meat
                   ½ fat

Chicken a La King
Serving Size: 5¼ ounces
Calories, 1 serving: 180
Exchange, 1 serving: ½ bread
                   1 lean meat
                   2 fat

CAMPBELL'S LOW-SODIUM PRODUCTS

Chicken Broth
Serving Size: 10½ ounces
Calories, 1 serving: 40
Exchange, 1 serving: 1 fat

Chicken with Noodles
Serving Size: 10¾ ounces
Calories, 1 serving: 160
Exchange, 1 serving: 1 bread
                   ½ lean meat

Chunky Beef & Mushroom
Serving Size: 10¾ ounces
Calories, 1 serving: 210
Exchange, 1 serving: 1½ bread
                   1½ lean meat
                   ½ fat

Chunky Vegetable Beef
Serving Size: 10¾ ounces
Calories, 1 serving: 170
Exchange, 1 serving: 1 vegetable
                   1 bread
                   1 lean meat
                   ½ fat

SWANSON FROZEN PRODUCTS—BREAKFAST

French Toast with Sausage
Serving Size: 6½ ounces
Calories, 1 serving: 450
Exchange, 1 serving: 2½ bread
                   2 lean meat
                   4 fat

Omelet with Cheese Sauce and Ham
Serving Size: 7 ounces
Calories, 1 serving: 400
Exchange, 1 serving: ½ bread
                   2½ lean meat
                   5 fat

Pancakes and Blueberry Sauce
Serving Size: 7 ounces
Calories, 1 serving: 400
Exchange, 1 serving: 1 fruit
4 bread
2 fat

SWANSON FROZEN PRODUCTS—ENTREES

Beef Enchilada
Serving Size: 1 Complete Entree
(11¼ ounces)
Calories, 1 serving: 440
Exchange, 1 serving: 3 bread
1½ lean meat
3½ fat

Fried Chicken
Serving Size: 1 Complete Entree
(7¼ ounces)
Calories, 1 serving: 390
Exchange, 1 serving: 2 bread
2 lean meat
3 fat

Fish 'n' Chips
Serving Size: 1 Complete Entree
(5 ounces)
Calories, 1 serving: 320
Exchange, 1 serving: 2 bread
1 lean meat
3 fat

Salisbury Steak
Serving Size: 1 Complete Entree
(5½ ounces)
Calories, 1 serving: 340
Exchange, 1 serving: 1½ bread
2 lean meat
3 fat

SWANSON FROZEN PRODUCTS—DINNERS

Bean and Beef Burrito
Serving Size: 1 Complete Dinner
(15¼ ounces)
Calories, 1 serving: 720
Exchange, 1 serving: 1 vegetable
5½ bread
2 lean meat
5 fat

Fried Chicken, Barbecue Flavored
Serving Size: 1 Complete Dinner
(9¼ ounces)
Calories, 1 serving: 560
Exchange, 1 serving: 1 vegetable
1 fruit
2½ bread
2½ lean meat
4½ fat

Beef
Serving Size: 1 Complete Dinner
(11½ ounces)
Calories, 1 serving: 320
Exchange, 1 serving: 1 vegetable
1 fruit
1½ bread
2½ lean meat
½ fat

Fried Chicken, Breast Portion
Serving Size: 1 Complete Dinner
(10¾ ounces)
Calories, 1 serving: 650
Exchange, 1 serving: 4 bread
3 lean meat
4½ fat

Lasagna
Serving Size: 1 Complete Dinner
      (13 ounces)
Calories, 1 serving: 410
Exchange, 1 serving: 1 vegetable
      1 fruit
      2½ bread
      ½ lean meat
      3 fat

Turkey
Serving Size: 1 Complete Dinner
      (11½ ounces)
Calories, 1 serving: 330
Exchange, 1 serving: 1 vegetable
      1 fruit
      1½ bread
      2½ lean meat
      ½ fat

SWANSON HUNGRY-MAN DINNERS

Chicken Parmigiana
Serving Size: 1 Complete Dinner
      (20 ounces)
Calories, 1 serving: 810
Exchange, 1 serving: 1 vegetable
      1 fruit
      2½ bread
      4 lean meat
      8 fat

Mexican
Serving Size: 1 Complete Dinner
      (22 ounces)
Calories, 1 serving: 920
Exchange, 1 serving: 1 vegetable
      6 bread
      2 lean meat
      8 fat

Chopped Beef Steak
Serving Size: 1 Complete Dinner
      (17½ ounces)
Calories, 1 serving: 600
Exchange, 1 serving: 1 vegetable
      1 fruit
      3 bread
      4 lean meat
      3½ fat

Western Style
Serving Size: 1 Complete Dinner
      (17½ ounces)
Calories, 1 serving: 750
Exchange, 1 serving: 1 fruit
      4 bread
      5 lean meat
      4 fat

SWANSON HUNGRY-MAN ENTREES

Beef Enchilada
Serving Size: 1 Complete Entree
      (16 ounces)
Calories, 1 serving: 660
Exchange, 1 serving: 4 bread
      2 lean meat
      6 fat

Fried Chicken, Dark Portions
Serving Size: 1 Complete Entree
      (11 ounces)
Calories, 1 serving: 620
Exchange, 1 serving: 3 bread
      4 lean meat
      5 fat

SWANSON MAIN COURSE ENTREES

Lasagna with Meat
Serving Size: 1 Complete Entree
      (13¼ ounces)
Calories, 1 serving: 450
Exchange, 1 serving: 1 vegetable
      3 bread
      2 lean meat
      2½ fat

Salisbury Steak
Serving Size: 1 Complete Entree
      (10 ounces)
Calories, 1 serving: 380
Exchange, 1 serving: 1½ bread
      3 lean meat
      2½ fat

Swanson Meat Pies
Serving Size: 1 Complete Pie
           (8 ounces)
Calories, 1 serving: 400
Exchange, 1 serving: 1 vegetable
                 2½ bread
                 1 lean meat
                 3½ fat

Turkey
Serving Size: 1 Complete Pie
           (8 ounces)
Calories, 1 serving: 430
Exchange, 1 serving: 1 vegetable
                 2½ bread
                 1 lean meat
                 4 fat

SWANSON HUNGRY-MAN MEAT PIES

Chicken
Serving Size: 1 Complete Pie
           (16 ounces)
Calories, 1 serving: 700
Exchange, 1 serving: 1 vegetable
                 4 bread
                 2½ lean meat
                 6 fat

Steak Burger
Serving Size: 1 Complete Pie
           (16 ounces)
Calories, 1 serving: 750
Exchange, 1 serving: 1 vegetable
                 4 bread
                 2½ lean meat
                 7 fat

SWANSON PLUMP AND JUICY

Chicken Cutlets
Serving Size: 3½ ounces
Calories, 1 serving: 230
Exchange, 1 serving: 1 bread
                 1½ lean meat
                 1½ fat

Chicken Drumlets
Serving Size: 3 ounces
Calories, 1 serving: 220
Exchange, 1 serving: 1 bread
                 1½ lean meat
                 1½ fat

Chicken Dipsters
Serving Size: 3 ounces
Calories, 1 serving: 220
Exchange, 1 serving: 1 bread
                 1½ lean meat
                 1½ fat

SWANSON LE MENU DINNERS

Beef Sirloin Tips
Serving Size: 1 Complete Dinner
           (11½ ounces)
Calories, 1 serving: 390
Exchange, 1 serving: 1 vegetable
                 1½ bread
                 4 lean meat
                 1 fat

Chicken a La King
Serving Size: 1 Complete Dinner
           (10¼ ounces)
Calories, 1 serving: 320
Exchange, 1 serving: 1 vegetable
                 1½ bread
                 2½ lean meat
                 1 fat

Chicken Cordon Bleu
Serving Size: 1 Complete Dinner
(11 ounces)
Calories, 1 serving: 460
Exchange, 1 serving: 1 vegetable
2½ bread
2½ lean meat
2½ fat

Ham Steak
Serving Size: 1 Complete Dinner
(9½ ounces)
Calories, 1 serving: 320
Exchange, 1 serving: 1 vegetable
2 bread
2 lean meat
1 fat

Sweet and Sour Chicken
Serving Size: 1 Complete Dinner
(11½ ounces)
Calories, 1 serving: 450
Exchange, 1 serving: 1 vegetable
1 fruit
2 bread
2 lean meat
3 fat

Carnation Products

Choc. Malted Milk
Serving Size: 3 heaping tsp.
Calories, 1 serving: 79
Protein, 1 serving: 1.1 g
Carbohydrates, 1 serving: 18.4 g
Fat, 1 serving: 0.8 g
Exchange, 1 serving: 1 bread

Nat'l Malted Milk
Serving Size: 3 heaping tsp.
Calories, 1 serving: 90
Protein, 1 serving: 3 g
Carbohydrates, 1 serving: 15.6 g
Fat, 1 serving: 1.7 g
Exchange, 1 serving: 1 bread
½ fat

Sugar Free Hot Cocoa Mix
Serving Size: 1 envelope
Calories, 1 serving: 79
Protein, 1 serving: 1.1 g
Carbohydrates, 1 serving: 18.4 g
Fat, 1 serving: 0.8 g
Exchange, 1 serving: ½ milk

Carnation Instant Breakfast (Vanilla)
Serving Size: 1 envelope
Calories, 1 serving: 70
Protein, 1 serving: 7 g
Carbohydrates, 1 serving: 9 g
Fat, 1 serving: 0 g
Exchange, 1 serving: ½ milk
1 bread
½ vegetable

**Carnation Instant Breakfast
(Strawberry)**
Serving Size: 1 envelope
Calories, 1 serving: 70
Protein, 1 serving: 7 g
Carbohydrates, 1 serving: 9 g
Fat, 1 serving: 0 g
Exchange, 1 serving: ½ milk
1 bread
½ vegetable

Carnation Instant Breakfast (Chocolate)
Serving Size: 1 envelope
Calories, 1 serving: 70
Protein, 1 serving: 7 g
Carbohydrates, 1 serving: 8 g
Fat, 1 serving: 1 g
Exchange, 1 serving: ½ milk
1 bread
½ vegetable

Carnation Instant Chocolate Malt
Serving Size: 1 envelope
Calories, 1 serving: 70
Protein, 1 serving: 7 g
Carbohydrates, 1 serving: 9 g
Fat, 1 serving: 1 g
Exchange, 1 serving: ½ milk
1 bread
½ vegetable

Dannon Products

Plain Yogurt
Serving Size: 8 oz. cup
Calories, 1 serving: 140
Protein, 1 serving: 10 g
Carbohydrates, 1 serving: 16 g
Fat, 1 serving: 4 g

Extra Smooth
Serving Size: 6 oz.
Calories, 1 serving: 190
Protein, 1 serving: 7 g
Carbohydrates, 1 serving: 33 g
Fat, 1 serving: 4 g

Flavored Yogurt
Serving Size: 8 oz. cup
Calories, 1 serving: 200
Protein, 1 serving: 10 g
Carbohydrates, 1 serving: 34 g
Fat, 1 serving: 3 g

Supreme
Serving Size: 6 oz.
Calories, 1 serving: 190
Protein, 1 serving: 6 g
Carbohydrates, 1 serving: 33 g
Fat, 1 serving: 4 g

Fruit-On-the-Bottom Yogurt
Serving Size: 8 oz. cup
Calories, 1 serving: 240
Protein, 1 serving: 9 g
Carbohydrates, 1 serving: 43 g
Fat, 1 serving: 3 g

Original Mini-Pack
Serving Size: 4.4 oz.
Calories, 1 serving: 130
Protein, 1 serving: 5 g
Carbohydrates, 1 serving: 23 g
Fat, 1 serving: 2 g

Hearty Nuts & Raisins
Serving Size: 8 oz.
Calories, 1 serving: 260
Protein, 1 serving: 11 g
Carbohydrates, 1 serving: 48 g
Fat, 1 serving: 3 g

Extra Smooth Mini-Pack
Serving Size: 4.4 oz.
Calories, 1 serving: 130
Protein, 1 serving: 5 g
Carbohydrates, 1 serving: 24 g
Fat, 1 serving: 2 g

Estee Products

Gelatin Desserts
Serving Size: ½ cup
Exchange, 1 serving: FREE
Calories, 1 serving: 8

Instant Puddings
Serving Size: ½ cup
Exchange, 1 serving: ½ milk,
                    ½ starch/bread
Calories, 1 serving: 70

Cake Mixes
Serving Size: ¹/₁₀th cake
Exchange, 1 serving: 1 starch/bread,
                    1 fat
Calories, 1 serving: 100

Frosting Mix
Serving Size: 1½ tsp.
Exchange, 1 serving: ¾ starch/bread
Calories, 1 serving: 50-60

Whipped Topping
Serving Size: 1 tbs.
Exchange, 1 serving: FREE
Calories, 1 serving: 4

Cookies
Serving Size: 2
Exchange: ½ starch/bread, ½ fat
Calories, 1 serving: 50

Duplex Sandwich Cookies
Serving Size: 3
Exchange, 1 serving: 1 starch/bread,
                    1½ fat
Calories, 1 serving: 120

Assorted Creme Wafers
Serving Size: 3
Exchange, 1 serving: 1 starch/bread,
                    1 fat
Calories, 1 serving: 90

Chocolate, Vanilla Creme Wafers
Serving Size: 3
Exchange, 1 serving: ½ starch/bread,
                    ½ fat
Calories, 1 serving: 60

Snack Wafers
Serving Size: 1
Exchange, 1 serving: ⅔ starch/bread,
                    1 fat
Calories, 1 serving: 80

Chocolate Coated Snack Wafers
Serving Size: 1
Exchange, 1 serving: 1 starch/bread,
                    1½ fat
Calories, 1 serving: 120

Salad Dressings
Serving Size: 1 tbs.
Exchange, 1 serving: FREE
Calories, 1 serving: 4-6

Dip Mixes
Serving Size: 2 tbs.
Exchange, 1 serving: 1 fat
Calories, 1 serving: 50

Mushroom Soup
Serving Size: 6 oz.
Exchange, 1 serving: ¼ milk
Calories, 1 serving: 30

Tomato Soup
Serving Size: 6 oz.
Exchange, 1 serving: ½ starch/bread
Calories, 1 serving: 40

Chicken Noodle Soup
Serving Size: 6 oz.
Exchange, 1 serving: ¼ milk, ¼ fat
Calories, 1 serving: 35

Manhattan Clam Chowder
Serving Size: 6 oz.
Exchange, 1 serving: 1 vegetable
Calories, 1 serving: 30

Beef Vegetable Soup
Serving Size: 6 oz.
Exchange, 1 serving: 1 vegetable
Calories, 1 serving: 30

Cocoa
Serving Size: 6 oz.
Exchange, 1 serving: ½ milk
Calories, 1 serving: 50

Brownie Mix
Serving Size: 2″×2″
Exchange, 1 serving: ½ starch/bread,
½ fat
Calories, 1 serving: 45

Unsalted Crackers
Serving Size: 2
Exchange, 1 serving: ½ starch/bread
Calories, 1 serving: 30

Unsalted Pretzels
Serving Size: 15
Exchange, 1 serving: 1 starch/bread
Calories, 1 serving: 75

6 Calorie Wheat Wafers
Serving Size: 6
Exchange, 1 serving: ½ starch/bread
Calories, 1 serving: 35

Wheat Snax
Serving Size: 1 oz.
Exchange, 1 serving: 1½ starch/bread
Calories, 1 serving: 110

Chocolate Bars
Serving Size: 2 squares
Exchange, 1 serving: ½ fruit, 1 fat
Calories, 1 serving: 60

Fruit and Nut Mix
Serving Size: 10 pieces
Exchange, 1 serving: ½ starch/bread,
1 fat
Calories, 1 serving: 85

Chocolate Coated Raisins
Serving Size: 10 pieces
Exchange, 1 serving: ½ starch/bread,
½ fat
Calories, 1 serving: 50

Peanut Butter Cups
Serving Size: 2
Exchange, 1 serving: ½ starch/bread,
1 fat
Calories, 1 serving: 90

Estee-ets
Serving Size: 8 pieces
Exchange, 1 serving: ½ starch/bread,
½ fat
Calories, 1 serving: 55

Gum Drops
Serving Size: 7
Exchange, 1 serving: ½ fruit
Calories, 1 serving: 20

Hard Candy
Serving Size: 2 pieces
Exchange, 1 serving: ½ fruit
Calories, 1 serving: 25

Lollipops
Serving Size: 1
Exchange, 1 serving: ¼ fruit
Calories, 1 serving: 12

Mints
Serving Size: 5
Exchange, 1 serving: ½ fruit
Calories, 1 serving: 20

Estee's Dia-Mel Products

Preserves and Jellies
Serving Size: 1 tsp.
Exchange, 1 serving: FREE
Calories, 1 serving: 2

Salad Dressings
Serving Size: 1 tbs.
Exchange, 1 serving: FREE
Calories, 1 serving: 1-2

Mayonnaise
Serving Size: 1 tbs.
Exchange, 1 serving: 3 fat
Calories, 1 serving: 106

Diet Whipped
Serving Size: 1 tbs.
Exchange, 1 serving: ½ fat
Calories, 1 serving: 24

Catsup
Serving Size: 1 tbs.
Exchange, 1 serving: FREE
Calories, 1 serving: 6

Peanut Butter
Serving Size: 2 tbs.
Exchange, 1 serving: 1 meat, 2 fat
Calories, 1 serving: 200

Pancake Syrup, Blueberry Syrup, Chocolate Syrup
Serving Size: 1 tbs.
Exchange, 1 serving: FREE
Calories, 1 serving: 1

Cake Mix
Serving Size: ¹/₁₀th cake
Exchange, 1 serving: 1 starch/bread,
1 fat
Calories, 1 serving: 100

Gelatin Desserts
Serving Size: ½ cup
Exchange, 1 serving: FREE
Calories, 1 serving: 8

Pancake Mix
Serving Size: 3′–3′
Exchange, 1 serving: 1½ starch/bread
Calories, 1 serving: 100

Vanilla, Chocolate, Butterscotch Puddings
Serving Size: ½ cup
Exchange, 1 serving: ½ milk
Calories, 1 serving: 50

Lemon Pudding
Serving Size: ½ cup
Exchange, 1 serving: ¼ fruit
Calories, 1 serving: 14

Ready-To-Eat Gel-a-thin
Serving Size: ½ cup
Exchange, 1 serving: FREE
Calories, 1 serving: 2

Beef Ravioli
Serving Size: 8 oz.
Exchange, 1 serving: 2¼ starch/bread,
½ meat, 1½ fat
Calories, 1 serving: 260

Spaghetti and Meatballs
Serving Size: 8 oz.
Exchange, 1 serving: 1½ starch/bread,
¾ meat, 1½ fat
Calories, 1 serving: 220

Chicken Stew
Serving Size: 8 oz.
Exchange, 1 serving: 1¼ starch/bread,
1 meat
Calories, 1 serving: 150

Beef Stew
Serving Size: 8 oz.
Exchange, 1 serving: 1¼ starch/bread,
2 meat
Calories, 1 serving: 200

Chili with Beans
Serving Size: 8 oz.
Exchange, 1 serving: 2 starch/bread,
2 meat, 2 fat
Calories, 1 serving: 360

Stuffed Dumplings
Serving Size: 8 oz.
Exchange, 1 serving: 1 starch/bread,
1 meat
Calories, 1 serving: 160

Tomato Soup
Serving Size: 8 oz.
Exchange, 1 serving: ¾ starch/bread
Calories, 1 serving: 50

Chicken Noodle Soup
Serving Size: 8 oz.
Exchange, 1 serving: ½ starch/bread,
¼ meat
Calories, 1 serving: 50

Cream of Mushroom Soup
Serving Size: 8 oz.
Exchange, 1 serving: ½ starch/bread,
                      1 fat
Calories, 1 serving: 85

Vegetable Beef Soup
Serving Size: 8 oz.
Exchange, 1 serving: 2 vegetable, ½ fat
Calories, 1 serving: 70

Picante Sauce
Serving Size: 2 tbs.
Exchange, 1 serving: ¼ vegetable
Calories, 1 serving: 8

Taco Sauce
Serving Size: 2 tbs.
Exchange, 1 serving: ½ vegetable
Calories, 1 serving: 14

Spaghetti Sauce
Serving Size: 4 oz.
Exchange, 1 serving: 1 vegetable,
                     1 fruit
Calories, 1 serving: 70

Steak Sauce
Serving Size: ½ oz.
Exchange, 1 serving: ½ vegetable
Calories, 1 serving: 15

Cocktail Sauce
Serving Size: 1 tbs.
Exchange, 1 serving: ¼ fruit
Calories, 1 serving: 10

Barbecue Sauce
Serving Size: 1 tbs.
Exchange, 1 serving: ½ fruit
Calories, 1 serving: 18

Health Valley Products

Real Granola-Al. Cr.-H.V.
Serving Size: 28 g
Calories, 1 serving: 120
Protein, 1 serving: 4 g
Carbohydrates, 1 serving: 20 g
Fat, 1 serving: 3 g

Real Granola-Haw Frt H.V.
Serving Size: 28 g
Calories, 1 serving: 120
Protein, 1 serving: 4 g
Carbohydrates, 1 serving: 20 g
Fat, 1 serving: 3 g

Swiss Brkfst/Tr Frt H.V.
Serving Size: 57 g
Calories, 1 serving: 200
Protein, 1 serving: 7 g
Carbohydrates, 1 serving: 37 g
Fat, 1 serving: 4 g

Swiss Brkfst/Rai Nut H.V.
Serving Size: 57 g
Calories, 1 serving: 200
Protein, 1 serving: 7 g
Carbohydrates, 1 serving: 37 g
Fat, 1 serving: 4 g

Chili-Mld Veg w/Bns H.V.
Serving Size: 113 g
Calories, 1 serving: 170
Protein, 1 serving: 9 g
Carbohydrates, 1 serving: 18 g
Fat, 1 serving: 7 g

Chili-Spcy Vet/Bns H.S.
Serving Size: 113 g
Calories, 1 serving: 170
Protein, 1 serving: 9 g
Carbohydrates, 1 serving: 18 g
Fat, 1 serving: 7 g

Soup—Beef Brth Ns Hlth Vly
Serving Size: 114 g
Calories, 1 serving: 10 g
Protein, 1 serving: 1 g
Carbohydrates, 1 serving: 2 g
Fat, 1 serving: 0 g

Soup—Clam Chowder Hlth Vly
Serving Size: 114 g
Calories, 1 serving: 80
Protein, 1 serving: 4 g
Carbohydrates, 1 serving: 8 g
Fat, 1 serving: 3 g

Soup—Minestrone Hlth Vly
Serving Size: 114 g
Calories, 1 serving: 90
Protein, 1 serving: 3 g
Carbohydrates, 1 serving: 10 g
Fat, 1 serving: 4 g

Soup—Potato Ns Hlth Vly
Serving Size: 114 g
Calories, 1 serving: 70
Protein, 1 serving: 3 g
Carbohydrates, 1 serving: 10 g
Fat, 1 serving: 2 g

Soup—Tomato Hlth Valley
Serving Size: 114 g
Calories, 1 serving: 60
Protein, 1 serving: 2 g
Carbohydrates, 1 serving: 8 g
Fat, 1 serving: 2 g

Soup—Chnky Splt Pea Ns H.V.
Serving Size: 114 g
Calories, 1 serving: 60
Protein, 1 serving: 4 g
Carbohydrates, 1 serving: 10 g
Fat, 1 serving: 1 g

Soup—Chnky Veg Beef H.V.
Serving Size: 114 g
Calories, 1 serving: 85
Protein, 1 serving: 4 g
Carbohydrates, 1 serving: 8 g
Fat, 1 serving: 4 g

Cheese Puffs/Ched Lts H.V.
Serving Size: 7 g
Calories, 1 serving: 40
Protein, 1 serving: 1 g
Carbohydrates, 1 serving: 4 g
Fat, 1 serving: 2 g

Pot Chps/Ctry Chps H.V.
Serving Size: 28 g
Calories, 1 serving: 160
Protein, 1 serving: 2 g
Carbohydrates, 1 serving: 14 g
Fat, 1 serving: 11 g

Pot Chps/Health Valley
Serving Size: 28 g
Calories, 1 serving: 160
Protein, 1 serving: 2 g
Carbohydrates, 1 serving: 14 g
fat, 1 serving: 11 g

Pretzl-Mini w/W H.V.
Serving Size: 28 g
Calories, 1 serving: 120
Protein, 1 serving: 4 g
Carbohydrates, 1 serving: 20 g
Fat, 1 serving: 2 g

Cookies/Ginger Snaps
Serving Size: 4 g
Calories, 1 serving: 15
Protein, 1 serving: 1 g
Carbohydrates, 1 serving: 2 g
Fat, 1 serving: 1 g

Cookie/Oatmeal Jumbo H.V.
Serving Size: 14 g
Calories, 1 serving: 60
Protein, 1 serving: 1 g
Carbohydrates, 1 serving: 10 g
Fat, 1 serving: 2 g

Cookie/Cinn Jumbo H.V.
Serving Size: 14 g
Calories, 1 serving: 60
Protein, 1 serving: 1 g
Carbohydrates, 1 serving: 10 g
Fat, 1 serving: 2 g

Crackers/Cheese Wheels H.V.
Serving Size: 28 g
Calories, 1 serving: 140
Protein, 1 serving: 4 g
Carbohydrates, 1 serving: 14 g
Fat, 1 serving: 7 g

Crackers/Herb Health Valley
Serving Size: 28 g
Calories, 1 serving: 130
Protein, 1 serving: 3 g
Carbohydrates, 1 serving: 16 g
Fat, 1 serving: 6 g

Crackers/Sesame Hlth Vly
Serving Size: 28 g
Calories, 1 serving: 130
Protein, 1 serving: 3 g
Carbohydrates, 1 serving: 16 g
Fat, 1 serving: 6 g

Crackers/Stnd Wht Hlth Vly
Serving Size: 28 g
Calories, 1 serving: 130
Protein, 1 serving: 3 g
Carbohydrates, 1 serving: 16 g
Fat, 1 serving: 6 g

Crackers/Sw Rye Hlth Vly
Serving Size: 28 g
Calories, 1 serving: 130
Protein, 1 serving: 3 g
Carbohydrates, 1 serving: 16 g
Fat, 1 serving: 6 g

Peanut Btr—Chunky Hlth Vly
Serving Size: 14 g
Calories, 1 serving: 83
Protein, 1 serving: 4 g
Carbohydrates, 1 serving: 3 g
Fat, 1 serving: 7 g

Peanut Btr—Crmy Hlth Vly
Serving Size: 14 g
Calories, 1 serving: 83
Protein, 1 serving: 4 g
Carbohydrates, 1 serving: 3 g
Fat, 1 serving: 7 g

Hodgson Mill Products

Hodgson Mill Cornbread & Muffin Mix
Serving Size: ⅞ oz. (1-3″ × 3″ piece)
Calories, 1 serving: 56
Protein, 1 serving: 2 g
Carbohydrates, 1 serving: 11 g
Fat, 1 serving: 3 g

Hodgson Mill Bran-Muffin Mix
Serving Size: 1.12 oz. (1 Lg. Muffin)
Calories, 1 serving: 129
Protein, 1 serving: 4 g
Carbohydrates, 1 serving: 21 g
Fat, 1 serving: 3.5 g

Hodgson Mill Whole Wheat Muffin Mix
Serving Size: 1.25 oz. (1 Lg. Muffin)
Calories, 1 serving: 140
Protein, 1 serving: 4 g
Carbohydrates, 1 serving: 23 g
Fat, 1 serving: 3 g

Hodgson Mill Buttermilk Biscuit Mix
Serving Size: ⅞ oz. (1 lg. biscuit)
Calories, 1 serving: 96
Protein, 1 serving: 2 g
Carbohydrates, 1 serving: 16 g
Fat, 1 serving: 2 g

Hodgson Mill Veggie Bows and Veggie Rotini
Serving Size: 2 oz. dry
Calories, 1 serving: 210
Protein, 1 serving: 7 g
Carbohydrates, 1 serving: 41 g
Fat, 1 serving: 1 g

Hodgson Mill Whole Wheat Macaroni & Cheese Dinner
Serving Size: 1.8 oz.
Calories, 1 serving: 207
Protein, 1 serving: 8 g
Carbohydrates, 1 serving: 43 g
Fat, 1 serving: less than 1 g

HODGSON MILL PASTAS

Whole Wheat Elbow Macaroni
Serving Size: 2 oz. dry
Calories, 1 serving: 230
Protein, 1 serving: 3 g
Carbohydrates, 1 serving: 48 g
Fat, 1 serving: less than 1 g

Cracked Wheat Cereal
Serving Size: ¼ cup (1.3 oz.)
Calories, 1 serving: 107
Protein, 1 serving: 3.8 g
Carbohydrates, 1 serving: 24 g
Fat, 1 serving: .66 g

Whole Wheat Medium Shells
Serving Size: 2 oz. dry
Calories, 1 serving: 230
Protein, 1 serving: 8 g
Carbohydrates, 1 serving: 48 g
Fat, 1 serving: less than 1 g

Whole Wheat Egg Noodles
Serving Size: 2 oz. dry
Calories, 1 serving: 220
Protein, 1 serving: 8 g
Carbohydrates, 1 serving: 40 g
Fat, 1 serving: 3 g

Whole Wheat Lasagna
Serving Size: 2 oz. dry
Calories, 1 serving: 230
Protein, 1 serving: 8 g
Carbohydrates, 1 serving: 48 g
Fat, 1 serving: less than 1 g

Pepperidge Farm Products

SPECIAL COLLECTION

Almond Supreme
Serving Size: 2 cookies
Calories, 1 serving: 140
Protein, 1 serving: 2 g
Carbohydrates, 1 serving: 13 g
Fat, 1 serving: 10 g

Milk Chocolate Macadamia
Serving Size: 2 cookies
Calories, 1 serving: 120
Protein, 1 serving: 2 g
Carbohydrates, 1 serving: 13 g
Fat, 1 serving: 7 g

Chocolate Chunk Pecan
Serving Size: 2 cookies
Calories, 1 serving: 130
Protein, 1 serving: 1 g
Carbohydrates, 1 serving: 15 g
Fat, 1 serving: 7 g

KITCHEN HEARTH COOKIES

Date Nut Granola
Serving Size: 3 cookies
Calories, 1 serving: 160
Protein, 1 serving: 1 g
Carbohydrates, 1 serving: 20 g
Fat, 1 serving: 9 g

Date Pecan
Serving Size: 3 cookies
Calories, 1 serving: 160
Protein, 1 serving: 1 g
Carbohydrates, 1 serving: 22 g
Fat, 1 serving: 8 g

Raisin Bran
Serving Size: 3 cookies
Calories, 1 serving: 160
Protein, 1 serving: 1 g
Carbohydrates, 1 serving: 20 g
Fat, 1 serving: 8 g

FRUIT COOKIES

Apricot-Raspberry
Serving Size: 3 cookies
Calories, 1 serving: 150
Protein, 1 serving: 1 g
Carbohydrates, 1 serving: 23 g
Fat, 1 serving: 6 g

Strawberry
Serving Size: 3 cookies
Calories, 1 serving: 150
Protein, 1 serving: 1 g
Carbohydrates, 1 serving: 23 g
Fat, 1 serving: 7 g

Blueberry
Serving Size: 3 cookies
Calories, 1 serving: 170
Protein, 1 serving: 2 g
Carbohydrates, 1 serving: 27 g
Fat, 1 serving: 6 g

THIN CRACKERS

Butter Flavored
Serving Size: 4 crackers
Calories, 1 serving: 80
Protein, 1 serving: 1 g
Carbohydrates, 1 serving: 10 g
Fat, 1 serving: 3 g

Cheese
Serving Size: 4 crackers
Calories, 1 serving: 70
Protein, 1 serving: 1 g
Carbohydrates, 1 serving: 8 g
Fat, 1 serving: 8 g

TINY GOLDFISH CRACKERS

Cheddar Cheese
Serving Size: 45 crackers
Calories, 1 serving: 140
Protein, 1 serving: 3 g
Carbohydrates, 1 serving: 18 g
Fat, 1 serving: 6 g

Pizza Flavored
Serving Size: 45 crackers
Calories, 1 serving: 140
Protein, 1 serving: 2 g
Carbohydrates, 1 serving: 18 g
Fat, 1 serving: 7 g

Parmesan Cheese
Serving Size: 45 crackers
Calories, 1 serving: 140
Protein, 1 serving: 3 g
Carbohydrates, 1 serving: 18 g
Fat, 1 serving: 6 g

Pretzel
Serving Size: 45 crackers
Calories, 1 serving: 120
Protein, 1 serving: 2 g
Carbohydrates, 1 serving: 21 g
Fat, 1 serving: 3 g

Original
Serving Size: 45 crackers
Calories, 1 serving: 140
Protein, 1 serving: 2 g
Carbohydrates, 1 serving: 18 g
Fat, 1 serving: 6 g

SNACK STICKS

Cheese
Serving Size: 8 crackers
Calories, 1 serving: 140
Protein, 1 serving: 3 g
Carbohydrates, 1 serving: 18 g
Fat, 1 serving: 6 g

Rye
Serving Size: 8 crackers
Calories, 1 serving: 130
Protein, 1 serving: 2 g
Carbohydrates, 1 serving: 20 g
Fat, 1 serving: 4 g

Original
Serving Size: 8 crackers
Calories, 1 serving: 130
Protein, 1 serving: 2 g
Carbohydrates, 1 serving: 20 g
Fat, 1 serving: 5 g

Sesame
Serving Size: 8 crackers
Calories, 1 serving: 130
Protein, 1 serving: 2 g
Carbohydrates, 1 serving: 18 g
Fat, 1 serving: 6 g

Pumpernickel
Serving Size: 8 crackers
Calories, 1 serving: 130
Protein, 1 serving: 2 g
Carbohydrates, 1 serving: 20 g
Fat, 1 serving: 5 g

DISTINCTIVE CRACKERS

English Water Biscuit
Serving Size: 4 crackers
Calories, 1 serving: 70
Protein, 1 serving: 1 g
Carbohydrates, 1 serving: 13 g
Fat, 1 serving: 1 g

Cracked Wheat
Serving Size: 4 crackers
Calories, 1 serving: 110
Protein, 1 serving: 2 g
Carbohydrates, 1 serving: 14 g
Fat, 1 serving: 4 g

Sesame
Serving Size: 4 crackers
Calories, 1 serving: 80
Protein, 1 serving: 2 g
Carbohydrates, 1 serving: 11 g
Fat, 1 serving: 3 g

Hearty Wheat
Serving Size: 4 crackers
Calories, 1 serving: 100
Protein, 1 serving: 2 g
Carbohydrates, 1 serving: 13 g
Fat, 1 serving: 4 g

Toasted Wheat with Onion
Serving Size: 4 crackers
Calories, 1 serving: 80
Protein, 1 serving: 3 g
Carbohydrates, 1 serving: 12 g
Fat, 1 serving: 3 g

FRUIT SQUARES

Apple
Serving Size: 1 square
Calories, 1 serving: 230
Protein, 1 serving: 1 g
Carbohydrates, 1 serving: 27 g
Fat, 1 serving: 12 g

Blueberry
Serving Size: 1 square
Calories, 1 serving: 230
Protein, 1 serving: 1 g
Carbohydrates, 1 serving: 29 g
Fat, 1 serving: 11 g

Cherry
Serving Size: 1 square
Calories, 1 serving: 230
Protein, 1 serving: 1 g
Carbohydrates, 1 serving: 29 g
Fat, 1 serving: 12 g

OLD FASHIONED MUFFINS

Apple with Spice
Serving Size: 1 muffin
Calories, 1 serving: 170
Protein, 1 serving: 3 g
Carbohydrates, 1 serving: 23 g
Fat, 1 serving: 8 g

Blueberry
Serving Size: 1 muffin
Calories, 1 serving: 180
Protein, 1 serving: 2 g
Carbohydrates, 1 serving: 27 g
Fat, 1 serving: 7 g

Bran with Raisin
Serving Size: 1 muffin
Calories, 1 serving: 180
Protein, 1 serving: 2 g
Carbohydrates, 1 serving: 28 g
Fat, 1 serving: 7 g

Carrot Walnut
Serving Size: 1 muffin
Calories, 1 serving: 170
Protein, 1 serving: 6 g
Carbohydrates, 1 serving: 27 g
Fat, 1 serving: 4 g

Chocolate Chip
Serving Size: 1 muffin
Calories, 1 serving: 200
Protein, 1 serving: 3 g
Carbohydrates, 1 serving: 28 g
Fat, 1 serving: 8 g

Cinnamon Swirl
Serving Size: 1 muffin
Calories, 1 serving: 190
Protein, 1 serving: 2 g
Carbohydrates, 1 serving: 30 g
Fat, 1 serving: 6 g

Corn
Serving Size: 1 muffin
Calories, 1 serving: 180
Protein, 1 serving: 3 g
Carbohydrates, 1 serving: 27 g
Fat, 1 serving: 7 g

Pillsbury Products

SWEET ROLLS

Pillsbury Soft Bread Sticks
Serving Size: 1 bread stick
Calories, 1 serving: 100
Protein, 1 serving: 3 g
Carbohydrates, 1 serving: 17 g
Fat, 1 serving: 2 g

Pillsbury Best Quick Cinnamon Rolls with Icing
Serving Size: 1 roll
Calories, 1 serving: 210
Protein, 1 serving: 2 g
Carbohydrates, 1 serving: 29 g
Fat, 1 serving: 9 g

Pillsbury Best Apple Danish with Icing
Serving Size: 1 roll
Calories, 1 serving: 240
Protein, 1 serving: 3 g
Carbohydrates, 1 serving: 33 g
Fat, 1 serving: 11 g

Pillsbury Cinnamon with Icing
Serving Size: 2 rolls
Calories, 1 serving: 230
Protein, 1 serving: 3 g
Carbohydrates, 1 serving: 34 g
Fat, 1 serving: 9 g

Hungry Jack Butter Tasting Cinnamon with Icing
Serving Size: 2 rolls
Calories, 1 serving: 290
Protein, 1 serving: 3 g
Carbohydrates, 1 serving: 37 g
Fat, 1 serving: 14 g

Pillsbury Orange Danish with Icing
Serving Size: 2 rolls
Calories, 1 serving: 290
Protein, 1 serving: 3 g
Carbohydrates, 1 serving: 39 g
Fat, 1 serving: 14 g

Pillsbury Cinnamon Raisin Danish with Icing
Serving Size: 2 rolls
Calories, 1 serving: 290
Protein, 1 serving: 3 g
Carbohydrates, 1 serving: 39 g
Fat, 1 serving: 14 g

Pillsbury Caramel Danish with Nuts
Serving Size: 2 rolls
Calories, 1 serving: 310
Protein, 1 serving: 4 g
Carbohydrates, 1 serving: 39 g
Fat, 1 serving: 16 g

PASTRIES

Pillsbury Apple Turnover
Serving Size: 1 turnover
Calories, 1 serving: 170
Protein, 1 serving: 2 g
Carbohydrates, 1 serving: 23 g
Fat, 1 serving: 8 g

Pillsbury Blueberry Turnovers
Serving Size: 1 turnover
Calories, 1 serving: 170
Protein, 1 serving: 2 g
Carbohydrates, 1 serving: 22 g
Fat, 1 serving: 8 g

Pillsbury Cherry Turnover
Serving Size: 1 turnover
Calories, 1 serving: 170
Protein, 1 serving: 2 g
Carbohydrates, 1 serving: 24 g
Fat, 1 serving: 8 g

COOKIES

Peanut Butter
Serving Size: 3 cookies
Calories, 1 serving: 200
Protein, 1 serving: 3 g
Carbohydrates, 1 serving: 28 g
Fat, 1 serving: 8 g

Sugar
Serving Size: 3 cookies
Calories, 1 serving: 200
Protein, 1 serving: 2 g
Carbohydrates, 1 serving: 30 g
Fat, 1 serving: 8 g

Chocolate Chip
Serving Size: 3 cookies
Calories, 1 serving: 210
Protein, 1 serving: 2 g
Carbohydrates, 1 serving: 29 g
Fat, 1 serving: 10 g

Oatmeal Raisin
Serving Size: 3 cookies
Calories, 1 serving: 200
Protein, 1 serving: 3 g
Carbohydrates, 1 serving: 28 g
Fat, 1 serving: 8 g

Fudge Brownies
Serving Size: 1 bar
Calories, 1 serving: 140
Protein, 1 serving: 1 g
Carbohydrates, 1 serving: 22 g
Fat, 1 serving: 5 g

PILLSBURY MICROWAVE FRENCH BREAD PIZZA

Cheese
Serving Size: 1 piece
Calories, 1 serving: 340
Protein, 1 serving: 14 g
Carbohydrates, 1 serving: 40 g
Fat, 1 serving: 14 g

Sausage and Pepperoni Combination
Serving Size: 1 piece
Calories, 1 serving: 430
Protein, 1 serving: 18 g
Carbohydrates, 1 serving: 41 g
Fat, 1 serving: 21 g

Pepperoni
Serving Size: 1 piece
Calories, 1 serving: 410
Protein, 1 serving: 17 g
Carbohydrates, 1 serving: 40 g
Fat, 1 serving: 20 g

Sausage
Serving Size: 1 piece
Calories, 1 serving: 410
Protein, 1 serving: 18 g
Carbohydrates, 1 serving: 40 g
Fat, 1 serving: 19 g

HEAT 'N EAT MICROWAVE PIZZA

Sausage
Serving Size: 4.8 ounces
Calories, 1 serving: 360
Protein, 1 serving: 13 g
Carbohydrates, 1 serving: 31 g
Fat, 1 serving: 20 g

Cheese
Serving Size: 4.1 ounces
Calories, 1 serving: 270
Protein, 1 serving: 13 g
Carbohydrates, 1 serving: 31 g
Fat, 1 serving: 11 g

Pepperoni
Serving Size: 4.6 ounces
Calories, 1 serving: 350
Protein, 1 serving: 13 g
Carbohydrates, 1 serving: 31 g
Fat, 1 serving: 18 g

Combination
Serving Size: 4.9 ounces
Calories, 1 serving: 380
Protein, 1 serving: 14 g
Carbohydrates, 1 serving: 31 g
Fat, 1 serving: 21 g

TOASTER STRUDEL BREAKFAST PASTRIES

Blueberry
Serving Size: 1 pastry
Calories, 1 serving: 190
Protein, 1 serving: 2 g
Carbohydrates, 1 serving: 28 g
Fat, 1 serving: 8 g

Apple Spice
Serving Size: 1 pastry
Calories, 1 serving: 190
Protein, 1 serving: 2 g
Carbohydrates, 1 serving: 28 g
Fat, 1 serving: 8 g

Cinnamon
Serving Size: 1 pastry
Calories, 1 serving: 190
Protein, 1 serving: 2 g
Carbohydrates, 1 serving: 26 g
Fat, 1 serving: 8 g

Cherry
Serving Size: 1 pastry
Calories, 1 serving: 190
Protein, 1 serving: 2 g
Carbohydrates, 1 serving: 26 g
Fat, 1 serving: 9 g

Raspberry
Serving Size: 1 pastry
Calories, 1 serving: 190
Protein, 1 serving: 2g
Carbohydrates, 1 serving: 27 g
Fat, 1 serving: 8 g

Strawberry
Serving Size: 1 pastry
Calories, 1 serving: 190
Protein, 1 serving: 2 g
Carbohydrates, 1 serving: 27 g
Fat, 1 serving: 8 g

TOASTER MUFFINS

Apple Spice Breakfast Muffins
Serving Size: 1 muffin
Calories, 1 serving: 140
Protein, 1 serving: 2 g
Carbohydrates, 1 serving: 24 g
Fat, 1 serving: 4 g

Banana Nut Breakfast Muffins
Serving Size: 1 muffin
Calories, 1 serving: 140
Protein, 1 serving: 2 g
Carbohydrates, 1 serving: 19 g
Fat, 1 serving: 6 g

Wild Main Blueberry Breakfast Muffins
Serving Size: 1 muffin
Calories, 1 serving: 130
Protein, 1 serving: 2 g
Carbohydrates, 1 serving: 22 g
Fat, 1 serving: 4 g

Old Fashioned Corn Breakfast Muffins
Serving Size: 1 muffin
Calories, 1 serving: 140
Protein, 1 serving: 3 g
Carbohydrates, 1 serving: 21 g
Fat, 1 serving: 5 g

Raisin Bran Breakfast Muffins
Serving Size: 1 muffin
Calories, 1 serving: 120
Protein, 1 serving: 2 g
Carbohydrates, 1 serving: 20 g
Fat, 1 serving: 4 g

TOTINO'S MICROWAVE PIZZAS

Sausage/Pepperoni Combination
Serving Size: 4.2 ounces
Calories, 1 serving: 310
Protein, 1 serving: 11 g
Carbohydrates, 1 serving: 31 g
Fat, 1 serving: 15 g

Pepperoni
Serving Size: 4 ounces
Calories, 1 serving: 290
Protein, 1 serving: 10 g
Carbohydrates, 1 serving: 31 g
Fat, 1 serving: 14 g

Sausage
Serving Size: 4.2 ounces
Calories, 1 serving: 300
Protein, 1 serving: 10 g
Carbohydrates, 1 serving: 31 g
Fat, 1 serving: 15 g

Cheese
Serving Size: 3.9 ounces
Calories, 1 serving: 250
Protein, 1 serving: 11 g
Carbohydrates, 1 serving: 31 g
Fat, 1 serving: 9 g

Index